Families and
Family Therapy

FAMILIES & FAMILY THERAPY

by Salvador Minuchin

HARVARD UNIVERSITY PRESS, CAMBRIDGE, MASSACHUSETTS

To my father and mother,
who taught me the meaning of families,
and to my wife and children,
who enlarged my experience.

Acknowledgments

This book owes a lot to an informal seminar that was held twice a day for thirty to forty minutes over more than two years as Jay Haley, Braulio Montalvo, and I were driving to and from the Philadelphia Child Guidance Clinic. Many of the ideas presented here emerged from our discussions, for which I am deeply grateful. I especially thank Braulio Montalvo, whom I consider my most influential teacher. He has the rare capacity to receive an idea and then give it back enlarged. At many times during our ten years of working together he has redirected my thinking, and has always enriched it. I have also benefited from the assistance of Frances Hitchcock, who for seven years helped me to clarify my ideas and to turn them into prose.

Many of my colleagues at the Philadelphia Child Guidance Clinic made contributions to this book, bouncing ideas back and forth with me. I especially want to mention the faculty of the Institute of Family Counseling, and in particular, Jerome Ford, Carter Umbarger, Marianne Walters, and Rae Weiner.

This book began as a series of lectures presented to groups in the United States, Sweden, and Holland. I wish to thank my students of the Group Psychotherapy Association in Holland, who contributed examples and shared their views. Mordecai Kaffman, M.D., kindly interviewed the Israeli family especially for this book. Finally, thanks are due to Lyman Wynne for his helpful suggestions in reviewing the manuscript and to Virginia LaPlante for her work in editing the book.

A NOTE ON THE TRANSCRIPTS

The transcripts in this book have been edited to protect the privacy of the families interviewed. When necessary, meanings have been clarified.

Before the presentation of the transcripts, references are sometimes made to the families involved, as examples of various points. This anticipatory device is used to familiarize the reader with the cases, so that when he reaches the full account of each session, he need give less attention to content and more to the therapeutic process.

The Smith, Dodds, and Gorden family interviews have been made into movies, with analysis provided by Braulio Montalvo. They are titled "I Think It's Me—Difference Display As a Contextual Event" (Chapter 9), "Affinity" (Chapter 10), and "A Family with a Little Fire" (Chapter 11). Information on these films is available from the Philadelphia Child Guidance Clinic, 1700 Bainbridge Street, Philadelphia, Pennsylvania 19146.

Salvador Minuchin, M.D.

Contents

1
Structural Family Therapy, 1

2
A Family in Formation: The
Wagners and Salvador Minuchin, 16

3
A Family Model, 46

4
A Kibbutz Family:
The Rabins and Mordecai
Kaffman, 67

5
Therapeutic Implications of a
Structural Approach, 89

6
The Family in Therapy, 110

7
Forming the Therapeutic
System, 123

8
Restructuring the Family, 138

9
A "Yes, But" Technique: The
Smiths and Salvador Minuchin, 158

10
A "Yes, And" Technique: The
Dodds and Carl A. Whitaker, 189

11
The Initial Interview: The Gordens
and Braulio Montalvo, 206

12
A Longitudinal View: The Browns
and Salvador Minuchin, 240

Epilog, 255

Further Readings, 259

Notes, 262

Index, 265

Families and
Family Therapy

1 Structural Family Therapy

Robert Smith, his wife, his twelve-year-old son, and his father-in-law are sitting with me for their first consultation with a family therapist. Mr. Smith is the identified patient. He has been hospitalized twice in the past seven years for agitated depression and has recently requested rehospitalization.

Minuchin: What is the problem? . . . So who wants to start?

Mr. Smith: I think it's my problem. I'm the one that has the problem. . .

Minuchin: Don't be so sure. Never be so sure.

Mr. Smith: Well . . . I'm the one that was in the hospital and everything.

Minuchin: Yeah, that doesn't, still, tell me it is your problem. Okay, go ahead. What is your problem?

Mr. Smith: Just nervous, upset all the time. . . seem to be never relaxed. . . I get uptight, and I asked them to put me in the hospital. . .

Minuchin: Do you think that you are the problem?

Mr. Smith: Oh, I kind of think so. I don't know if it is caused by anybody, but I'm the one that has the problem.

Minuchin: . . . Let's follow your line of thinking. If it would be caused by somebody or something outside of yourself, what would you say your problem is?

Mr. Smith: You know, I'd be very surprised.

1

Minuchin: Let's think in the family. Who makes you upset?
Mr. Smith: I don't think anybody in the family makes me upset.
Minuchin: Let me ask your wife. Okay?

The consultation that began with this exchange was the beginning of a new approach to the problem of Mr. Smith. Instead of focusing on the individual, the therapist focused on the person within his family. The therapist's statement, "Don't be so sure," challenged the certainty that Mr. Smith alone was the problem or had the problem—a certainty which had been shared by Mr. Smith, his family, and the many mental health professionals he had encountered.

The therapist's framework was structural family therapy, a body of theory and techniques that approaches the individual in his social context. Therapy based on this framework is directed toward changing the organization of the family. When the structure of the family group is transformed, the positions of members in that group are altered accordingly. As a result, each individual's experiences change.

The theory of family therapy is predicated on the fact that man is not an isolate. He is an acting and reacting member of social groups. What he experiences as real depends on both internal and external components. The paradoxical duality of the human perception of reality is explained by Ortega y Gasset in a parable: "Peary relates that on his polar trip he traveled one whole day toward the north, making his sleigh dogs run briskly. At night he checked his bearings to determine his latitude and noticed with great surprise that he was much further south than in the morning. He had been toiling all day toward the north on an immense iceberg drawn southwards by an ocean current."[1] Human beings are in the same situation as Commander Peary on the iceberg. Man's experience is determined by his interaction with his environment.

To say that man is influenced by his social context, which he also influences, may seem obvious. Certainly the concept is not new; it was familiar to Homer. But it is a new approach to base mental health techniques on this concept.

The traditional techniques of mental health grew out of a fascination with individual dynamics. This preoccupation dominated the field and led therapists to concentrate on exploring the intrapsychic. Of necessity, the resulting treatment techniques focused exclusively on the individual, apart from his surroundings. An artificial "boundary" was drawn between the individual and his social context.

In theory, this boundary was recognized as artificial, but in practice it was maintained by the process of therapy. As the patient was treated in isolation, the data encountered were inevitably restricted to the way he alone felt and thought about what was happening to him; such individualized material in turn reinforced the approach to the individual apart from his context and provided little possibility for corrective feedback. The very richness of the data available discouraged other approaches. As a result, the individual came to be viewed as the site of pathology.

A therapist oriented to individual therapy still tends to see the individual as the site of pathology and to gather only the data that can be obtained from or about the individual. For instance, an adolescent boy might be referred to therapy because he is shy and daydreams in class. He is a loner, with difficulty relating to his peers. A therapist who operates in individual sessions would explore the boy's thoughts and feelings about his present life and the people in it, the historical development of his conflict with parents and siblings, and the compulsive intrusion of this conflict into extrafamilial, seemingly unrelated situations. He would establish contact with the family and the school, but to understand the boy and the boy's relationship with his family, he would rely mainly on the content of the boy's communication and on transferential phenomena. An internal cognitive-affective rearrangement is regarded as the necessary step to facilitate improvement of the presenting problem.

A therapist working within this framework can be compared to a technician using a magnifying glass. The details of the field are clear, but the field is severely circumscribed. A therapist working within the framework of structural family therapy, however, can be compared to a technician with a zoom lens. He can zoom in for a closeup whenever he wishes to study the intrapsychic field, but he can also observe with a broader focus.

If the same boy were referred to a family therapist, the therapist would explore his interactions within significant life contexts. In family interviews, the therapist would observe the relationship of the boy and his mother, with its mingled closeness and hostility. He might see that when the boy talks in the presence of his parents, he rarely addresses his father, or that when he does talk to his father, he tends to do so through his mother, who translates and explains her son to her husband. He might notice that other siblings seem more spontaneous, interrupt the parents, and talk to the father and mother alike. Thus, the therapist does not have to depend on the boy's descriptions of his father, mother, and siblings to postulate the introjection of the familial figures. The family members are present, demonstrating behavior in relation to the boy that can be operationally described. The broader focus and the greater flexibility opened to the therapist enhance the possibilities for therapeutic intervention. The therapist is not restricted to the family interaction as internalized by the boy, but can himself experience the way in which the family members support and qualify each other. He then develops a transactional theory to explain the phenomena he is observing. He can also be in touch with the boy's school, since the presenting problem is related to school performance, and the theories and techniques of family therapy lend themselves readily to work with the individual in contexts other than the family.

Thus, the family therapist does not conceive of an "essential" personality, remaining unchanged throughout the vicissitudes of different contexts and circumstances. He sees the boy as a member of different social contexts, acting and reacting within them. His concept of the site of pathology is much broader, and so are the possibilities for intervention.

MAN IN HIS CONTEXT

Structural family therapy, approaching man in his social context, was developed in the second half of the twentieth century. It is one of many responses to the concept of man as part of his environment that began to gain currency early in the century. Individual psychodynamic thinking drew upon a different concept, that of man as a hero, remaining himself in spite of circumstances. An example of this concept appears in *Paradise Lost*. When Satan is defeated in his revolt against God and cast into hell, he defies his circumstances:

> The mind is its own place, and of itself
> Can make a Heav'n of Hell, a Hell of Heav'n.[2]

This perception of the individual could survive in a world where the resources of man seemed infinite. Modern technology has changed this view. The earth no longer appears as a limitless territory, waiting for its claimant, but as a spaceship whose resources are dwindling. These changes are reflected in man's current perceptions of himself and of his way of being.

As early as 1914, Ortega y Gasset wrote: "I am myself plus my circumstances, and if I do not save it, I cannot save myself. This sector of circumstantial reality forms the other half of my person; only through it can I integrate myself and be fully myself. The most recent biological science studies the living organism as a unit composed of the body and its particular environment so that the life process consists not only of the adaptation of the body to its environment, but also of the adaptation of the environment to its body. The hand tries to adjust itself to the material object in order to grasp it firmly; but at the same time, each material object conceals a previous affinity with a particular hand."[3] There is a striking similarity between this poetic observation at the beginning of the century and the more modern explanation, couched in cibernetic language, with which Gregory Bateson erased the boundary between inner and outer space to achieve his own metaphor of the mind: "Consider a man felling a tree with an axe. Each stroke of the axe is modified or corrected, according to the shape of the cut face of the tree left by the previous stroke. This self-corrective ... process is brought about by a total system, tree-eyes-brain-muscles-axe-stroke-tree; and it is this total system that has the characteristics of ... mind."[4] The old idea of the individual acting upon his environment has here become the concept of the individual interacting with his environment. To paraphrase Ortega, a man is not himself without his circumstances.

Bateson's metaphor of the mind and Ortega's poetic imagery of man and his circumstances are corroborated by experiments, which have demonstrated that context directly influences the internal processes of the mind. For example, the neurologist José Delgado, who experimented with the implantation of electrodes in animals' brains, showed conclusively that while an animal responds to the triggering effect of electrical stimulation, the behavior thus triggered is organized by the animal's context. Writing of his experiments with monkeys, he reported: "It is well known that monkey colonies constitute autocratic societies in which one animal establishes itself as boss of the group, claiming a large portion of the territory, feeding first, and being avoided by the others, who ... express their submissiveness. ... In several colonies we have observed that radio stimulation ... in the boss monkey increased his aggressiveness and induced well-directed attacks against other members of the group, whom he chased around and occasionally bit. ... It was evident that his hostility was oriented purposefully ... because he usually attacked the other male who represented a challenge to his authority, and he always spared the little female who was his favorite partner."[5] In other words, the internal, electrical triggering of behavior was always modified by the context. The electrical stimulation could produce aggression, but the expression of that aggression was related to the social group.

Delgado's interest in the relationship between electrical stimulation of the brain and the social context of the stimulated animal led him to experiment with changing the animal's social context. The social rank of a female monkey was altered by changing the composition of the group. In the first group she was the lowest of four, in the second group she was ranked third, and in the third group she was ranked second. In all three colonies, the electrical stimulations induced the monkey to run across her cage, climb, lick, vocalize, and attack other animals. In the first group, she tried to attack another monkey only once. In group two she became more aggressive, attacking twenty-four times. In group three, the stimulated monkey attacked other monkeys seventy-nine times. Delgado concluded: "intraspecies aggression has been evoked ... by electrical stimulation of several cerebral structures, and its expression is dependent on the social setting ... an artificially evoked aggressive act may be directed against a specific group member or may be entirely suppressed, according to the stimulated subject's social rank."[6]

Delgado also found that if a low-ranking monkey is mildly stimulated in the rage center, he may not show a rage response at all. This finding might be explained as repression. But it is also possible to explain the monkey's lack of response in terms of two different inputs, one of which is more powerful. If the input of the low-ranking monkey's context is more powerful than the stimulation of the brain, rage might not be felt. If the stimulation is increased, the monkey's behavior within its context changes, as it does if the social circumstances are changed.

Delgado carries his observations further into a consideration of the influence of the social sphere on man. "We cannot be free from parents, teachers, and society," he wrote, "because they are the extracerebral sources of our minds."[7] Delgado's concept of cerebral and extracerebral mind is directly comparable to Bateson's and Ortega's concepts.[8] A human mind develops as the brain processes and stores the multiple inputs triggered both internally and externally. Information, attitudes, and ways of perceiving are assimilated and stored, thereby becoming part of the person's approach to the current context with which he interacts.

The family is a highly significant factor in this process. It is a natural social group, which governs its members' responses to inputs from within and without. Its organization and structure screen and qualify family members' experience. In many cases, it can be seen as the extracerebral part of the mind.

The influence of the family on its members was demonstrated experimentally by an investigation of childhood psychosomatic illness being conducted by myself, Lester Baker, and our team. The research findings provided experimental grounding for the basic tenet of family therapy, namely, that the child responds to stresses affecting the family. We developed a method of measuring individual physiological responses to family stress. During a structured family interview designed for this purpose, blood samples are drawn from each family member in such a way that obtaining the samples does not interfere with ongoing interactions. The level of plasma-free fatty acids in the samples is later analyzed. Free fatty acid (FFA) is a biochemical indicator of emotional arousal—the concentration rises within five to fifteen minutes of emotional stress. By comparing the FFA levels at different times during the structured interview, the individual's response to family stress can be physiologically documented.

The FFA results of the Collins family are a good example (Figure 1). Both children were diabetics. Dede, 17, had had diabetes for three years; her sister Violet, 12, had been diabetic since infancy. Studies of

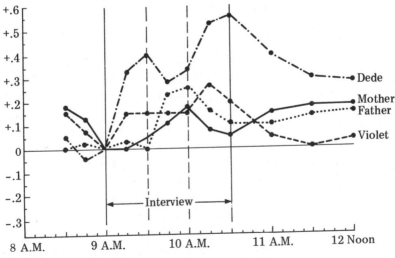

Fig. 1. Change in Free Fatty Acid, the Collins family

the children's "physiological lability" showed that there was no obvious difference in their individual responsivity to stress. Yet these two children, with the same metabolic defect, having much of the same genetic endowment, and living in the same household with the same parents, presented very different clinical problems. Dede was a "superlabile diabetic"; that is, her diabetes was affected by psychosomatic problems. She was subject to bouts of ketoacidosis that did not respond to insulin administered at home. In three years, she had been admitted to the hospital for emergency treatment twenty-three times. Violet had some behavioral problems that her parents complained of, but her diabetes was under good medical control.

During the interview designed to measure the children's response to stress, lasting from 9 to 10 A.M., the parents were subjected to two different stress conditions, while the children watched them through a one-way mirror. Although the children could not take part in the conflict situation, their FFA levels rose as they observed their stressed parents. The cumulative impact of current psychological stress was powerful enough to cause marked physiological changes even in children not directly involved. At 10 o'clock the children were brought into the room with their parents. It then became clear that they played very different roles in this family. Dede was trapped between her parents. Each parent tried to get her support in the fight with the other parent, so that Dede could not respond to one parent's demands without seeming to side against the other. Violet's allegiance was not sought. She could therefore react to her parents' conflict without being caught in the middle.

The effects of these two roles can be seen in the FFA results. Both children showed significant increments during the interview, between 9 and 10, and even higher increments between 10 and 10:30, when they were with their parents. After the end of the interview at 10:30, however, Violet's FFA returned to baseline promptly. Dede's remained elevated for the next hour and a half.

In both spouses, the FFA levels increased from 9:30 to 10, indicating stress in the interspouse transactions. But their FFA decreased after the children had come in to the room and the spouses had assumed parental functions. In this family, interspouse conflict was reduced or detoured when the spouses assumed parental functions. The children functioned as conflict-detouring mechanisms. The price they paid is shown by both the increase in their FFA levels and Dede's inability to return to baseline. The interdependence between the individual and his family—the flow between "inside" and "outside"—is poignantly demonstrated in the experimental situation, in which behavioral events among family members can be measured in the bloodstream of other family members.

THE SITE OF PATHOLOGY

When the mind is viewed as extracerebral as well as intracerebral, to locate pathology within the mind of the individual does not indicate whether it is inside or outside the person. Pathology may be inside the patient, in his social context, or in the feedback between them. The artificial boundary becomes blurred, and therefore the approach to pathology must change. Therapy designed from this point of view rests on three axioms. Each has an emphasis quite different from the related axiom of individual theory. First, an individual's psychic life is not entirely an internal process. The individual influences his context and is influenced by it in constantly recurring sequences of interaction. The individual who lives within a family is a member of a social system to which he must adapt. His actions are governed by the characteristics of the system, and these characteristics include the effects of his own past actions. The individual responds to stresses in other parts of the system, to which he adapts; and he may contribute significantly to stressing other members of the system. The individual can be approached as a subsystem, or part, of the system, but the whole must be taken into account. The second axiom underlying this kind of therapy is that changes in a family structure contribute to changes in the behavior and the inner psychic processes of the members of that system. The third axiom is that when a therapist works with a patient or a patient family, his behavior becomes part of the context. Therapist and family join to form a new, therapeutic system, and that system then governs the behavior of its members.

These three assumptions—that context affects inner processes, that changes in context produce changes in the individual, and that the therapist's behavior is significant in change—have always been part of the common sense basis of therapy. They have occupied the background in the literature of psychotherapy, while internal processes have come to the fore. However, they have not become central to psychotherapeutic practice, where an artificial dichotomy between the individual and his social context still exists.

An example can be drawn from concepts of paranoid thinking,

because in this area an understanding of the patient's context is vital. Yet in intrapsychic terms, paranoia is approached as a formal thinking disorder, in which the perception of events is determined by internal processes. As Aaron Beck wrote: "among normals, the sequence perception-cognition-emotion is dictated largely by the demand character of the stimulus situation. . . [However] the paranoid patient may selectively abstract those aspects of his experience that are consistent with his preconceived idea of persecution, etc. He may make arbitrary judgments which have no factual basis. These are usually manifested by reading hidden significances and meanings into events. He also tends to overgeneralize isolated instances of intrusion, discrimination, etc."[9] In these terms, paranoia is an internal phenomenon only tangentially related to reality.

Contrast this with a context-related view of paranoia. In a study of mental patients with paranoid symptoms, Erving Goffman pointed out that in early stages of the illness, the social context enters a complementarity with the patient which supports his illness.[10] Significant social groups, such as job peers, try to contain the patient, because his symptoms have a disruptive effect. They avoid him when possible and exclude him from decisions. They employ a humoring, pacifying, noncommittal style of interaction, which dampens the patient's participation as much as possible. They may even spy on him or form a collusive net so as to inveigle him into receiving psychiatric attention. Their well-meant tact and secrecy deprive the patient of a corrective feedback, with the ultimate consequence of constructing around the paranoid a real paranoid community.

Paranoid thinking and behavior can also be created experimentally in normal, highly educated professionals by group experiences, such as those devised at the Leadership Institutes of the Tavistock Clinic. In the "large-group exercise," thirty to fifty participants are seated in three to five concentric circles. The faculty are scattered through the circles, wearing business clothes, poker-faced, and silent. The group is given an ambiguous task: to study its own behavior.

Within the structure of this leaderless exercise, participants make statements that are not directed to anyone in particular, and because of the seating arrangements, half the participants have their backs turned and cannot see who is speaking. Dialog does not develop; a statement may be followed by a different statement in a different area. Thus, communications are not validated by consenting or dissenting feedback. Again and again, one sees the rapid appearance of suspicion, confusion about the nature of reality that is being experienced, the search for a target, and finally, the appearance of scapegoats in the group or the labeling of the faculty as omnipotent persecutors. In this context, "paranoid thinking" invariably develops in and is expressed by participants whose life circumstances and developmental histories have otherwise been very diverse.[11] It is thus clear that individual experience depends on the individual's idiosyncratic characteristics in his current life context.

A CASE STUDY

In Wonderland, Alice suddenly grew to a gigantic size. Her experience was that she got bigger while the room got smaller. If Alice had grown in a room that was also growing at the same rate, she might have experienced everything as staying the same. Only if Alice or the room changes separately does her experience change. It is simplistic, but not inaccurate, to say that intrapsychic therapy concentrates on changing Alice. A structural family therapist concentrates on changing Alice within her room.

The treatment of a patient with paranoid thought disorders is instructive of these different views. An Italian widow in her late sixties, who had lived in the same apartment for twenty-five years, came home one day to find the apartment robbed. She decided to move and called a moving company. It was the beginning of a nightmare. As she described it, the people who came to move her things tried to control where she went. When they moved her belongings, they purposely misplaced and lost precious possessions. They left sinister markings—cryptograms—on her furniture. When she went outside, people followed her, secretly signaling to each other. She went to a psychiatrist, who gave her tranquillizers, but her experiences did not change. She was then referred to an inpatient unit, where another psychiatrist interviewed her. He purposely left bottles on the table. Although she did not know what they were, they appeared clearly dangerous to her. He recommended hospitalization, but she refused.

She went to see another therapist, whose interventions were based on an ecological understanding of the old and lonely. He explained to the woman that she had lost her shell—the previous home where she had known each object, the neighborhood, and the people in the neighborhood. At this point, like any crustacean that has lost its shell, she was vulnerable. Reality had a different experiential effect. These problems would disappear, he assured her, when she grew a new shell. They discussed how to shorten the time this would take. She was to unpack all her belongings, hang up the pictures that had decorated her previous apartment, put the books on the shelves, and organize the apartment so that it became familiar. All her movements were to be routinized. She was to get up at a certain time, shop at a certain time, go to the same stores, the same checkout counters, and so on. She was not to try to make new friends in the new neighborhood for two weeks. She was to go back to visit her old friends, but in order to spare her friends and family, she was not to describe any of her experiences. If anyone inquired about her problems, she was to explain that they were merely the problems of illogical, fearful old people.

This intervention established a routine to help the patient increase her sense of familiarity with a new territory, in much the way that animals explore and examine a strange area. The frightening experience of unfamiliarity with new circumstances had been interpreted by this lonely person as a conspiracy against her. In the very measure by which she had tried to communicate her experiences, her environmental feedback had amplified her experience of being abnormal and psychotic. Her relatives and friends had become frightened for her and had in turn frightened her by their conspiracy of secrecy. A paranoid community had developed around her. Two psychiatrists diagnosed her condition as a psychosis with a paranoid delusion and, in accordance with that interpretation, proposed seclusion.

A context-related therapist, however, interpreted the movement to a new apartment as an ecological crisis. Following the metaphor of Alice in her room, he perceived the woman as changing more slowly than her world. His intervention involved changing the position of the woman in her world by giving her control over her world until it had become familiar. He moved in to protect the woman by taking over the situation, guiding her while she "grew a new shell." At the same time he blocked the feedback processes that were amplifying the patient's pathology. As his intervention changed the patient's experience of her circumstances, her symptoms disappeared rapidly. She continued living in her new apartment, with the independence she desired. In this example, as in the parable of Commander Peary, the change occurred not so much inside or outside the patient as in the way that the patient related to her circumstances.

Structural family therapy deals with the process of feedback between circumstances and the person involved—the changes imposed by a person on his circumstances and the way in which feedback to these changes affects his next move. A shift in the position of a person vis-à-vis his circumstances constitutes a shift of his experience. Family therapy uses techniques that alter the immediate context of people in such a way that their positions change. By changing the relationship between a person and the familiar context in which he functions, one changes his subjective experience.

For example, a twelve-year-old girl had asthma, which was psychosomatically triggered. She was on heavy medication, missed school often, and in the previous year had to be taken to the emergency room three times. She was referred to a child psychiatrist, who insisted on seeing the entire family—two parents and the identified patient's two older siblings. During the first interview, the therapist directed the family's attention to the oldest girl's obesity. The family's concern then shifted to include worry about the newly identified patient. The asthmatic child's symptoms then diminished to the point that her asthma was controllable on considerably less medication, and she stopped losing school time.

Change had taken place in the structure of the family. It moved from two parents protectively concerned with one child's asthma to two parents concerned with one child's asthma and another child's obesity. The previously identified patient's position in the family had changed and, concomitantly, her experience changed. She began to see her older sister as a person also having difficulties. Her parents' concerned and overprotective way of interacting with her diminished with the addition of another target of concern. The therapist had changed part of the family's organization in such a way as to make movement possible. He joined them in a modality familiar to them—concern—but amplified the target of concern. The new perspective changed the experience of the family members.

This is the foundation of family therapy. The therapist joins the family with the goal of changing family organization in such a way that the family members' experiences change. By facilitating the use of alternative modalities of transaction among family members, the therapist makes use of the family matrix in the process of healing. The changed family offers its members new circumstances and new perspectives of themselves vis-à-vis their circumstances. The changed organization makes possible a continuous reinforcement of the changed experience, which provides a validation of the changed sense of self.

The individual is not ignored in this theoretical structure. The individual's present is his past plus his current circumstances. Part of his past will always survive, contained and modified by current interactions. Both his past and his unique qualities are part of his social context, which they influence as the context influences him. What comes out of studies like Delgado's is a respect for the individual in his context, a concern not only with the individual's inherent and acquired characteristics but also with his interaction in the present. Man has memory; he is the product of his past. At the same time, his interactions in his present circumstances support, qualify, or modify his experience.

Structural family therapy utilizes this framework of conceptualizing man in his circumstances. The target of intervention could as well be any other segment of the individual's ecosystem that seems amenable to change-producing strategies.

THE SCOPE OF THE THERAPIST

The scope of the family therapist and the techniques he uses to pursue his goals are determined by his theoretical framework. Structural family therapy is a therapy of action. The tool of this therapy is to modify the present, not to explore and interpret the past. Since the past was instrumental in the creation of the family's present organization and functioning, it is manifest in the present and will be available to change by interventions that change the present.

The target of intervention in the present is the family system. The therapist joins that system and then uses himself to transform it. By changing the position of the system's members, he changes their subjective experiences.

To this end the therapist relies on certain properties of the family system. First, a transformation in its structure will produce at least one possibility for further change. Second, the family system is organized around the support, regulation, nurturance, and socialization of its members. Hence, the therapist joins the family not to educate or socialize it, but rather to repair or modify the family's own functioning so that it can better perform these tasks. Third, the family system has self-perpetuating properties. Therefore, the processes that the therapist initiates within the family will be maintained in his absence by the family's self-regulating mechanisms. In other words, once a change has been effected, the family will preserve that change, providing a different matrix and altering the feedback which continuously qualifies or validates family members' experiences.

These concepts of structure are the foundation of family therapy. However, structural family therapy must start with a model of normality against which to measure deviance. Interviews with effectively functioning families from different cultures will illustrate the normal difficulties of family life, which transcend cultural differences.

2 A Family in Formation: The Wagners and Salvador Minuchin

The family is a social unit that faces a series of developmental tasks. These differ along the parameters of cultural differences, but they have universal roots. This common aspect of family situations was ably expressed by Giovanni Guareschi:

Why do I keep talking about myself, about Margherita, and Albertino, and the Pasionaria? There is, truly, nothing "exceptional" about us ... Margherita is not an "unusual" woman. Neither are Albertino and the Pasionaria "extraordinary" children.

There are a hundred different varieties of grape—from white to black, from sweet to sour, from small to large. But if you press a hundred bunches of grapes of different varieties, the juice is always wine. If you squeeze grapes, you never get gasoline, milk, or lemonade.

And it's the juice that counts—in everything.

And the juice of my family is the same as the juice of millions of "ordinary" families, because the basic problems of my family are the same as those of millions of families: they spring from a family situation based on the necessity of adhering to the principles that are the foundation of all "ordinary" homes.[1]

The Wagners, in the interview that follows, are an ordinary family; that is, the couple has many problems of relating to one another, bringing up children, dealing with in-laws, and coping with the outside world. Like all normal families, they are constantly struggling with these problems and negotiating the compromises that make a life in common possible.

The interview with them was conducted to illustrate the stages and processes of family development. As the Wagners are a young family, the session was directed toward the exploration of family formation and of the changes that occur in a family with the arrival of the first child.

A number of tasks face a young couple at the beginning of marriage. The spouses must develop a mutual accommodation in a large number of small routines. For example, they must develop routines for going to bed and getting up at approximately the same time. There must be a routine for having meals together, and for setting and clearing the table. There must be a routine for being naked and for having sex, for sharing the bathroom and the Sunday paper, for watching the television and selecting the programs, and for going out together to places that both of them enjoy.

In this process of mutual accommodation, the couple develops a set of patterned transactions—ways in which each spouse triggers and monitors the behavior of the other and is in turn influenced by the previous behavioral sequence. These transactional patterns form an invisible web of complementary demands that regulate many family situations.

The couple also faces the task of separating from each family of origin and negotiating a different relationship with parents, siblings, and in-laws. Loyalties must shift, for the new spouses' primary commitments are to their marriage. The families of origin must accept and support this break.

In the same way, encounters with the extrafamilial—work, duties, and pleasures—must be reorganized and newly regulated. Decisions must be reached as to how the demands of the outside world will be allowed to intrude on the life of the new family. Each spouse must meet the other's friends and select those who are to become the couple's friends. Each spouse may gain new friends and lose touch with old ones.

The birth of a child marks a radical change in the family organization. The spouses' functions must differentiate to meet the infant's demands for care and nurturance and to handle the constraints thus imposed on the parents' time. The physical and emotional commitment to the child usually requires a change in the spouses' transactional patterns. A new set of subsystems appears in the family organization, with children and parents having different functions. This period also requires a renegotiation of boundaries with the extended family and the extrafamilial. Grandparents, aunts, and uncles may enter to support, guide, or organize the new functions in the family. Or the boundary around the nuclear family may be strengthened.

Children become adolescents and then adults. New siblings join the family, or the parents become grandparents. At different periods of development, the family is thus required to adapt and restructure. Changes in the relative strength and productivity of family members require continual accommodation, as does the general change from the children's dependency on their parents to the parents' dependency on their children. As children leave the family, the original unit of husband and wife reappears, but in very different social circumstances. The family must meet the challenge of both internal and external change while maintaining its continuity, and must support and encourage all its members' growth while adapting to a society in transition. These tasks are not easy.

The couple in this interview illustrate some of the difficulties. Emily and Mark Wagner were married four years ago. They have one son, Tommy, aged three. A year ago they went to a marriage counselor for four sessions. Now they label themselves as a normal family that has struggled through difficulties. They are proud of having reached a level of development at which there is mutual support and growth.

They answered an advertisement in a local newspaper asking for a normal family to participate in an interview in return for a fee. The interview was conducted before a large audience of family therapists, who were sitting in the same room and responding to the interview as it unfolded. Tommy was in the room playing with a babysitter.

The interview is not a therapeutic interview. It is a developmental interview, designed to gather historical material and to elicit the participants' perceptions of their family's functioning. In an interview with a normal family, there is an implicit contract. The family, having labeled itself normal at the start, will be confirmed and supported in this belief by the interview. When it leaves, it will still consider itself to be a normal family.

Minuchin: The first thing that I want to know is why are you here? How did you resolve to do it? What was the process?

Mr. Wagner: Saturday, as far as I'm concerned, is our free day, so to speak. Whatever she would like to do, well then, we should do. I'm willing to go along with it. Sunday, then, is more or less my day.

Minuchin: That's an interesting thing; that means that you decide to divide the weekend in terms of days in which you make the major decisions and days in which your wife does?

Mr. Wagner: Not quite, it's sort of a—

Minuchin: It just happens. How did that happen? That's interesting historically; how did you come to this kind of division of decision making? Do you remember?

Mr. Wagner: I will hazard to venture a guess. I used to work Mondays through Saturdays, in the hospital business; Saturday was sort of bat-around. I felt Sunday was my day off, as far as I was concerned. So as soon as Saturday was available, she jumped at it, so to speak. I wouldn't let her have her preference on Sunday, because Sunday was sort of my day.

Minuchin: So, you evolved that kind of implicit rule without ever having it stated that this is the way you function.

Mrs. Wagner: As a rule, on Sunday he goes fishing or something, and I go my way. It's always been that way; well, it's been that way for about a year.

Minuchin: He goes fishing Sunday. Saturday is the day on which both of you do things together, and you are the one that decides.

Mr. Wagner: It's not, it's not that hard and fast, really. I would say that on Saturday there is a better chance that my wife would decide what we are going to do.

Mrs. Wagner: I usually have something planned, you know, that I want to do, and we usually do it.

The Wagners are discussing a transactional pattern that has evolved in the course of their married life. Although they are able to reconstruct the development of this pattern and do not consider it "hard and fast," it is nevertheless a rule that has become part of the arrangement of their life in common. Emily Wagner "usually has something planned" for Saturday, and they "usually" do it. On Sundays, each spouse pursues his own activities. Both spouses would consider an unnecessary infringement of this pattern as a personal betrayal. Moral and emotional components accompany contractual transactional patterns, even those whose origins and reasons have been lost.

Minuchin: How did it happen in this situation? Your wanting to come here?

Mrs. Wagner: To come here? I saw an ad in the paper and called up about it. My mother saw an ad in the paper.

Minuchin: Your mother? What about your family? Do they live around you?

Mrs. Wagner: They live in the same community.

Mr. Wagner: We are going to my place tomorrow, to my parents' house.

Minuchin: Do your parents live nearby?

Mr. Wagner: An eighth of a mile.

Minuchin: And your parents?

Mrs. Wagner: Oh, I'd say about three or four miles.

Minuchin: How important are your mother and father?

Mr. Wagner: I would say that—

Mrs. Wagner: Not much, really.

Mr. Wagner: No, not to the extent that her parents are.

Mrs. Wagner: Both his parents are working, and as a rule we don't see his parents that much when they are working, and Sunday is their only day to do things that they have to do. We don't see them as often as we see mine, but then again, we don't see mine that often, either. He doesn't; I do more, during the week.

Minuchin: That means Emily's family is involved with your family more centrally than Mark's. Was that in the beginning before Tommy came?

Mr. Wagner: I would say so.

Mrs. Wagner: We lived with my parents before Tommy came, when we first got married.

Minuchin: When you married, you moved to your parents'?

Mrs. Wagner: He was still in college. He was at the university at the time, finishing out a semester there. And so we stayed there. We lived with them from April until August. And it was horrible.

Minuchin: Your family didn't want him?

Mrs. Wagner: They wanted him, but they thought that—we started dating each other when we were sixteen. I was sixteen, he was seventeen, so when we first started dating each other there wasn't anything said until, oh, I think when we got pinned.

Minuchin: How old were you when you married?

Mrs. Wagner: Nineteen.

Minuchin: And your parents invited you to go with them?

Mrs. Wagner: They just said come live with us, until we went to Kansas.

Minuchin: You just decided that this was the only solution that you had, you didn't have alternatives there?

Mr. Wagner: Well, we could have lived outside, but my still being in school, I didn't want to drop out of school; I wanted to continue full time, so the only way we could afford this would be to reduce our housing costs as much as possible, so we accepted. We could have moved outside, but under the circumstances, we did accept their offer, so that we could save—so that we were really not captive, it wasn't a matter of being forced to live there; it was a matter of economics. We just decided we would live with it until we could return.

Minuchin: What happened then? Here you are, coming from two families, joining together, and wanting to create your own thing, but go to live to your family—how did that work? You said you lived there for how long? Six months?

Mrs. Wagner: Four months. I think I resented more or less not being in my own apartment and everything; I just felt like I couldn't, I really couldn't be a wife.

Minuchin: Why couldn't you be a wife?

Mrs. Wagner: Oh, I can't explain it; it's just a woman's feeling I had.

Mr. Wagner: No, I think perhaps I can say a little bit about it. It was resentment of her father. Her father tends to be the type that likes to make very strong suggestions as to what course of action I take in just about anything. I found that I could easily accept or reject and he wouldn't become upset about it, so that as far as I was concerned, it didn't concern me. She, however, because of these emotional feelings that she built up towards her father, any suggestion he made, she just rejected it completely and resented the fact that he was forever making suggestions here, there, and everywhere.

Minuchin: Well, let me see if I understand what Mark said in a different way. It seems to me that you married and you (*to wife*) wanted a separation from the family. You wanted to create a boundary and he was supposed to help you create the boundary. Now you lived in your home and Mark was getting along with your parents. Did he support—did he help you to increase the boundaries around you being a wife, or did he become a son of your parents?

Mrs. Wagner: I don't know if I can answer that.

Minuchin: Were you angry at him sometimes when he palled with your father, when you were angry with your father? When he palled with your mother when you were angry with your mother?

Mrs. Wagner: No, he never took sides, as far as—

Minuchin: It's impossible.

Mr. Wagner: I didn't really take sides—

Minuchin: It's impossible.

Mrs. Wagner: He didn't—he never came out and said, "You're wrong." And it usually—it was me. It was not my family. It was me.

Minuchin: Look, if he didn't take sides, he was taking sides.

Mrs. Wagner: He kept his mouth shut, though.

Minuchin: That was taking sides. You know, because, didn't you expect him to take your side?

Mrs. Wagner: Oh yes, but—

Minuchin: So, if he didn't take it, he was taking the opposite side.

Mrs. Wagner: But if he had opened his mouth, there would have been more trouble.

Minuchin: If he did not attack your mother when you attacked her, then he was siding with your mother, even if he didn't do anything.

Mr. Wagner: Umm hum.

When two partners join with the intention of forming a family, this is the formal beginning of a new family unit. But there are many steps between the formal initiation of a family and the creation of a viable unit. One of the tasks a new couple faces is the negotiation of their relationship with each spouse's family of origin. In addition, each family of origin must adjust to the separation or partial separation of one of its members, the inclusion of a new member, and the assimilation of the spouse subsystem within the family system's functioning. If the long-established structures of the families of origin do not change, they may threaten the processes of forming the new unit.

Minuchin: How did it work, really? With whom did you have the arguments? With your father or with your mother?

Mrs. Wagner: My mother—no! I don't know. I can't remember.

Mr. Wagner: Your father through your mother.

Mrs. Wagner: Was it that way? I can't remember, it's been so long.

Minuchin: He said, "Your father through your mother." That's a nice way of putting it. Is that the way in which it works?

Mr. Wagner: It's not completely related to her mother and her father; part of the problems were me. I always felt that my mother-in-law and I were in a sense a buffer zone between them. I always felt that if I thought my wife was wrong, I could tell her, and if she was completely wrong, I would say, "You're wrong," but if I didn't feel she was entirely wrong, I—I might have felt that she was wrong in what she did, but that there might have been some kind of a reason for it, at least as far as she was concerned.

Minuchin: Is Mark always logical?

Mrs. Wagner: Ummm hummm.

Minuchin: Well, that must be very painful.

Mrs. Wagner: At times. He's very logical and I'm completely illogical. We're as different as night and day.

Minuchin: So that during this period you wanted to be a wife and you were still a daughter.

Mrs. Wagner: Right.

Minuchin: And they didn't grow up. Your parents didn't grow up.

Mrs. Wagner: Not my—no, I wouldn't say it was my parents; I would say it was me.

Minuchin: No, they didn't grow up either.

Mrs. Wagner: Oh, I think I disagree with you.

Minuchin: They continued treating you as a daughter at a point at which you were a wife.

Mrs. Wagner: Maybe they did. Yeah, I guess that's it.

Minuchin: You know? That means that they didn't grow up. In terms of you, in terms of this new situation, they continued treating you as a daughter when you were now somebody different. You were a daughter, but you were a wife.

Mrs. Wagner's parents were unable to change to adapt to changed circumstances. Instead of learning to treat her as a wife, involved in the formation of a new social unit, they continued to treat her chiefly as their daughter, leaving her new husband in the difficult position of having to choose between his wife and his mother-in-law. The situation the Wagners are describing is a "boundary" problem—a problem of negotiating appropriate rules for the formation of new subsystems. It is also a problem of inappropriately maintaining transactional patterns.

Minuchin: What's your first name?

Mrs. Wagner: Emily.

Minuchin: Emily. Okay, my name is Sal. What kind of family is your family? Maybe you can describe your family. And Mark can help you, but only if you need it. Okay? You start first, and maybe if she needs you, Mark, she will call.

Mrs. Wagner: Well, I have a brother that I didn't speak to up until about three years ago. We fought like cats and dogs. I have a close relationship with my mother. My father, I couldn't stand until I got married. And that's about it.

Minuchin: That doesn't seem to be too close.

Mrs. Wagner: No, but then there's a whole, there's a closeness in some degree, you know, and there's permanence in other degrees.

Minuchin: Were they very controlling? Were they concerned about your movement?

Mrs. Wagner: Well, my father, yes, and my mother, no. My mother was very lenient; she used to cover up for the things that I did wrong.

Minuchin: Umph. So there was something between you, your father, and your mother in which you could play one against the other.

Mrs. Wagner: Well, but I—I smoked at thirteen. I didn't have permission from my father until I was sixteen, and yet I was allowed to smoke in front of my mother. When he was out, I would burn the house down.

Minuchin: That's quite a triangle.

Mrs. Wagner: I used to play sick, you know, stay home from school, and she knew I wasn't sick after about 8:15, and she'd cover up for me to stay out the rest of the day.

Mr. Wagner: Oh, something a little further than that—

Minuchin: Wait a moment. She is describing her family and she is supposed to ask you.

Mrs. Wagner: He wants to get in his thing.

Mr. Wagner: I know as an example, later on, when we knew each other, if we were out until 2:00 or 3:00 at night, if Papa knew, whew— the house would rumble, but he never knew.

Mrs. Wagner: Your mother and father never knew, either.

Mr. Wagner: No, they didn't care, though, that's the difference.

Minuchin: In your family, something was going on between your father and your mother in which you joined your mother.

Mrs. Wagner: I remember one incident, I don't know what it was, my father got mad at something. I was, you know, fresh; I had a terrible mouth and thought nothing of telling him to get off my back. I must have been maybe fifteen, I don't even know what it was that I got him upset about, but I know that he wasn't speaking to me because he was furious over something I did, and my mother let me go out because she didn't agree with his theory there, and he didn't speak to her for the rest of the day, he was so aggravated. I mean that was the type of situation, just one incident—

Minuchin: So your mother was fighting your father through you.

Mrs. Wagner: Probably, yeah. Ah, I can't remember my father ever hitting me until I was about fifteen, and then he did. I think he struck me once. He struck me a couple of times, and that did it; I didn't speak to him. And he told his brother that—I was very arrogant. I had no respect for him.

Minuchin: I am interested in moving both of you through the ways in which a family develops, so we started with your family and what I think is a triangle in which your mother fostered your anger at your father. Let's go to your family, Mark. What kind of family was it? I want you to understand what I am trying to do. I want to know some of the things that you need to create in order to separate from your families of origin.

Mr. Wagner: Well, I can start with the differences, between the two. My family in contrast is extremely close. I have a brother and sister and we are all very close. It might be due to the fact that my parents were very definitely together.

Minuchin: How many brothers do you have?

Mr. Wagner: An older brother and a younger sister. We've always done things together, with very little dissension or fighting of this nature within the family.

Mrs. Wagner: I think you're wrong there. You know your mother—

Minuchin: Wait a moment, do you want to let her in?

Mr. Wagner: Yeah, okay.

Mrs. Wagner: You and your mother carry on as though you are close, but your father is an outside member—

Mr. Wagner: Yeah, he's sort of a Johnny-come-lately in a sense. My mother was the guiding torch of the family.

Minuchin: Big torch or little torch?

Mr. Wagner: Little torch—about this big (*laughs*).

Minuchin: But his father was outside?

Mrs. Wagner: His father had nothing to do with the family, really. His mother was the guide; I mean, she made the decisions; she did everything for the children.

Mr. Wagner: She took care of all my clothing and socially and just about in every way. This is true. Or was—has been—true. Without going into a lot of detail, the only person that wasn't perhaps close, not that close, was my father. He was the only person that was perhaps a little different in that he wasn't part of the unit. At the present, though, that whole situation has changed. At that time, though, he was an outsider. There wasn't that much strife, because we just tried to avoid each other in a sense.

Minuchin: You and your father.

Mr. Wagner: Yeah, I would just—just avoid him. I actually did the same with her father if I disagreed with him.

Minuchin: In disagreement you avoid them?

Mr. Wagner: If I disagreed with him, I would avoid him, so to speak. I would just disregard his wish if I didn't think it was fair. If I thought it was fair, I would abide by it, my mother always sided with him, anyway.

Minuchin: Your mother would side with your father?

Mr. Wagner: Yes, I would say she backed him up in many bad decisions—she really went out of her way. If it was very out of line, however, she would always rationalize for him, and try to make us understand why.

Each spouse has now described the functioning of the parental subsystem in each family of origin. The parental subsystem is the unit of the family that bears the main responsibility for guiding and nurturing the children.

In Emily Wagner's family of origin, the parental subsystem was the middle class norm, a husband and wife couple. But husband and wife conflicts spilled over into the arena of parenting. Parental authority was split, and each parent attacked the other spouse through their daughter. The mother encouraged her to disobey the father; the father attacked her when he was angry at his wife. In Mark Wagner's family of origin, the parents had agreed to a distribution of functions. The mother carried out most of the nurturing tasks and the father was rather peripheral. But the children experienced their mother as representing their father's authority.

Minuchin: So you came to develop a family, and each of you had a model of how to talk. You know, there were some rules that Mark learned, and some rules that Emily learned, and these rules apparently were different.

Mr. Wagner: That's right.

Minuchin: Okay, now, you went together, and what happened? You needed to create your own rules. How did that develop?

When partners join, each expects the transactions of the spouse unit to take the forms with which he is familiar. Each spouse will try to organize the spouse unit along lines that are familiar or preferred, and will press the other to accommodate. A number of arrangements are possible. Each spouse will have areas in which he cannot permit flexibility. In other areas, alternative ways of relating can be chosen in response to the other's preferences. Each spouse will confirm the other in some situations and disqualify him in others. Some behaviors are reinforced and others are shed as the spouses accommodate to and assimilate each other's preferences. In this way, a new family system is formed.

Minuchin: How were the first years? The first year of marriage, what happened?

Mrs. Wagner: It stank.

Minuchin: He lets you say the affective thing, you know? So you say it stank. How was it for you, Mark?

Mr. Wagner: Ah, it was a disappointment to a degree, because—not any more or less than I really expected it to be, in a way.

Minuchin: Oh, that's a lot of crap.

Mr. Wagner: Yeah, it was. Because I knew, when we got married, that we couldn't buy a house.

Minuchin: Yeah, but that's nothing. That's not the way in which—in which you experience—

Mr. Wagner: I went into it a little more romantically than that. I was certain that it would be overcome easily.

Minuchin: Is he always an understater of things? You said it stank, and he said with his logical—

Mrs. Wagner: He is logical in everything. He rationalizes what I was telling you, even though he might really not feel that way—

Minuchin: You mean, probably, the same thing. It's just different ways of saying exactly the same thing. If I would translate what he said to your language, you know what I would say?

Mrs. Wagner: What?

Minuchin: It stank. Do you want to say how it stank, or do you want Mark to do it?

Mrs. Wagner: No, we know how it stank (*laughs*). Put two immature people in a room together and naturally it's going to stink.

Minuchin: But in different ways.

Mrs. Wagner: Well, he was a student, so he had, when things got bad, Mark could go to his books. And he'd really plug, and when things got bad, I'd sit there and drum on him and make a mountain out of—they really got blown out of proportion, and I think if I hadn't had Tommy, I probably would have left him after the first month of being trapped.

Minuchin: Who?

Mrs. Wagner: Tommy, my son. If I hadn't had him, I probably would have packed my bags and gone running home to mother after the first month of being with him alone. I'd say the second month. The first month was all right; we were still unpacked—

Minuchin: No, but you said the first four months you—

Mrs. Wagner: Oh, this is when we moved out.

Minuchin: Okay, that means that's—the first four months it stank in one way and then it stank in a different way.

Mrs. Wagner: Right. It stank for 2½ years.

Mr. Wagner: It had more downs—

Mrs. Wagner: It had more downs than it had ups.

Minuchin: And probably you thought that that was unique in your situation.

Mrs. Wagner: Unique? I thought it was horrible.

Minuchin: Okay, so, how did it work, then? He—what were you studying?

Mr. Wagner: Biology and business—biology, initially.

Minuchin: Where was that?

Mr. Wagner: City College, Kansas.

Minuchin: Okay, so what happened then? He would withdraw and he would go to his books.

Mrs. Wagner: Right.

Minuchin: And you didn't have anything to do.

Mrs. Wagner: I'd sit there and talk.

Minuchin: Could you take him out of the books? Could you talk with him?

Mrs. Wagner: If I got him mad enough, he'd fight back, but he's easygoing and he has to reach a boiling point before he really loses his temper.

Mr. Wagner: Emily, I think you're misunderstanding him. (*To Minuchin*) I think you are talking about our ability to communicate.

Minuchin: I am talking about how it stank.

Mr. Wagner: This was in essence the problem, communications.

Mrs. Wagner: We didn't communicate.

Mr. Wagner: There were very serious differences of opinion (*laughs*) about many things, one of which was living in Kansas, ah—initially you hated it—

Mrs. Wagner: I think if we had lived anyplace, for the first 2½ years it would have been the same.

Mr. Wagner: Well, probably that was just your way of expressing it, just Kansas. She didn't like the way we were living; she didn't care for the fact that I was going to school; she wanted a little bit more, initially, I think.

Mrs. Wagner: We didn't communicate at all. There was no communication at all between us for two years. After the lunge, you know, "I hate you" and "I hate you"—that was the extent of our communications. We finally got to a point that we hated each other after a while.

Mr. Wagner: Or we thought we did.

Mrs. Wagner: You know what it was? He could escape and I didn't have any way to escape, so I would just sit there.

Minuchin: Of course. He really didn't change too much his way of living. He was a student before; he was a student after. In what way did life change for you?

Mrs. Wagner: There was nothing, except you have to wait to have a baby and then have the baby and take care of him.

Minuchin: What did you do before you married?

Mrs. Wagner: I was a student, and then I worked for a while.

Minuchin: Thus, Mark's style of life was not disrupted by marriage, and yours was.

Mrs. Wagner: Pardon me, I'm sorry, I didn't understand that.

Minuchin: Your style of life was very disrupted by the marriage. His style was not.

Mrs. Wagner: Right, I think so; I think you could say that.

Minuchin: And so you wanted more from him.

Mrs. Wagner: Yeah, in that he was continuing his same routine that he had been continuing before we got married.

Minuchin: He didn't recognize that he was married.

Mrs. Wagner: I think he recognized that—well, he did in a certain degree. He came home to an apartment that was clean and meals—I think after Tommy came, there was a little bit more disruption (*laughs*).

Minuchin: Okay. Let's not bring in Tommy yet. You moved away after a terrible four months, when you were still a daughter when you were a wife; then you moved out to Kansas. And there you were not a daughter any more, because your parents were not there; you were not a student; you were not working; but in some way or another, you were not a wife.

Mrs. Wagner: I guess you could say that, yeah.

A marriage must replace certain social arrangements that have been given up for the formation of the new unit. Creation of the new social system means the creation or strengthening of a boundary around the couple. They are separated from certain former contacts and activities. The investment in the marriage is made at the expense of other relationships.

The degree of investment in the marriage may depend on how much has been given up. Mark Wagner kept the same job, studying, when he and Emily went to Kansas. She was cut off from her former life, however, so that she demanded much more of the relationship than Mark did.

Minuchin: Now, what did you do to change that?

Mrs. Wagner: What do you mean, now?

Minuchin: No, then. You see, because I can understand that for Mark it was easier to be married without changing really too much of his previous commitment. But it was very different for you. It was up to you, then, to try to change it, because he was comfortable. What did you do?

Mrs. Wagner: What did I do?

Minuchin: Yeah, how did you—how did you shake him up? You see, he was asleep.

Mrs. Wagner: Oh, I don't know, I can't—

Minuchin: How did she shake you up? (*Long pause.*)

Mr. Wagner: You've only seen one side of the story (*laughs*). Ah, no, as I see it, she didn't try to shake me up, really. What she did was stop communicating, altogether.

Mrs. Wagner: Ummm.

Mr. Wagner: See, I couldn't even talk to her. She just didn't want to discuss anything.

Mrs. Wagner: I built a big wall around myself.

Minuchin: That's a way of communicating. You were saying to him—

Mrs. Wagner: Get lost—

Minuchin: Well, or change.

Mrs. Wagner: I think it was me that had to change, though. I think

it was more or less I had to change. I was immature. I went into
marriage with the wrong idea—

Minuchin: He was immature also!

Mrs. Wagner: Right! He had—

Minuchin: He was not married, you see?

Mrs. Wagner: But see, I didn't, I didn't realize this at the time. I just
took anything that happened and blamed it on myself—

Minuchin: Why?

Mrs. Wagner: Because I usually instigated things—I mean, he would
be very quietly, you know, writing a term paper or something—

Minuchin: That's his style—his style is an understater—you were the
one who would need to activate something if you want to get on him,
but he made you feel guilty.

Mrs. Wagner: I would say it was fifty-fifty. I would make myself feel
guilty, and then he would go along with me and say, "You are a
bitch," you know, and back me right up.

Minuchin: Mark, when did you become married? I think, Emily,
that because you moved away, you really needed him and you were
more committed to this marriage than he was in the beginning.

Mrs. Wagner: Yes.

Minuchin: So, Mark, when did you become married?

Mr. Wagner: About a year ago (*laughs*).

Minuchin: Okay, let's follow this. You know, I just want to tell you
that what you are saying is very common, you know. I would say that
probably beats the laws of chance. You know, it is specific for each
couple. But all couples go through things like that. And some never,
never become married, you see. So the process from the *rite du pas-
sage* that you had with the justice of the peace, or whatever it is, to
the point of being married can really go for a very, very long time.
Some people divorce without ever really having been married.

Mrs. Wagner: Oh, we thought about that, too, I mean—

Mr. Wagner: I realized that, even then, that something had to
change, but then I tried to rationalize, "Well, what's the problem?"
(*Laughs.*) "Okay. We'll go to the source—what are the sources of the
problem?" Well, obviously, an adjustment is necessary on both parts.
For me, it's a very simple adjustment, because it's for all intents
and purposes very little different. No change whatsoever. In her case,
I knew it was a radical change. You see this was where I was wrong.
You see, I was too much in my own rut at my own speed. I had to
keep on just as I was, really plugging away. The barrier was there and

I really didn't try to break it down; I would try to make the attempt, nothing happened, I would go back to my own way, saying that sooner or later I was going to iron myself out, or when the situation changes, I'm going to iron myself out—when we move away—when I'm out of school, etc. And it did, but I don't think it did for that particular reason. I think it did because I matured myself and realized that there was a lot more giving involved than I had done.

The task of establishing the Wagner family took a rather long time, partly because the couple was embedded in social situations that handicapped the formation of a viable spouse unit. First they lived with Emily's parents. Emily had been part of a dysfunctional transactional pattern in her parents' marriage. When she married, they were unable to relinquish her, and they even drew her husband into their accustomed pattern. Mark and Emily were unable to support each other in strengthening the boundary between themselves and her parents. When they moved away, Mark's needs as a student and as a partial breadwinner engaged him, leaving him with little capacity for significant emotional involvement with his wife. Patterns of mutual support were overwhelmed by dysfunctional patterns.

Minuchin: Let's think what happened at this point. You know, at this point something major happened. When was Tommy born?
Mrs. Wagner: After we went to Kansas.
Minuchin: Now what happened?
Mrs. Wagner: It didn't get any better. It got worse.
Minuchin: Okay, how? Now you had Tommy.
Mrs. Wagner: Right, so I didn't need Mark. I just shut him out completely, you know.
Minuchin: You became a mother.
Mrs. Wagner: Right.
Minuchin: What happened to you?
Mr. Wagner: I didn't change enough, probably. I did change somewhat, but again, I was behind my little wall.
Minuchin: Was Tommy significant for you?
Mr. Wagner: Oh, yes.
Mrs. Wagner: We had a very close—when—at the time of his birth it was very close; I mean, well, he stayed with me through the labor.
Minuchin: Did you, did you have natural child birth?
Mr. Wagner: Not really, I wasn't with her through the delivery. I was with her through labor and up to delivery.

Minuchin: Now, she had Tommy and she did not need you, so what happened to you?

Mrs. Wagner: Nothing. He kept studying.

Mr. Wagner: Nothing really changed. In a sense, to me—

Mrs. Wagner: He went to classes the same night that his son was born in the morning. He was in classes though he hadn't been in bed all night.

Minuchin: Oh. So what happened? You see, now something new had happened. She had a child of her own. She was a mother. And you could be a father or you could not be, you know? You had an alternative.

When a child is born, new functions must appear. The functioning of the spouse unit must be modified to meet the demands of parenting. In general, the system must make the complex changes required to shift from a system of two to a system of three.

Usually the woman's commitment to a unit of three, including a deeper commitment to the marriage, begins with pregnancy. The child is a reality for her much earlier than for the man. He begins to feel like a father only at the birth, and sometimes even later than that. The man may remain uncommitted while the woman is already adapting to a new level of family formation.

Mrs. Wagner: He's always been a father.

Mr. Wagner: I don't really know what to say. I can't think now—and I can't say that I changed, you know, radically, or a major change. Of course, I was delighted to have a son. As she says, perhaps the relationship between Emily and me had not improved any. It might even have gotten worse.

Minuchin: Why?

Mr. Wagner: Nevertheless we did have one bond, and we both loved our child. I guess I would have to say that in a conventional way I was delighted and I was excited and it added something to the family.

Minuchin: But she was—she changed in relationship to you.

Mr. Wagner: She had said that after the birth of the baby, Tommy, things got worse. Now this is something—I realize that there was continuous strife there and unhappy feelings, but I didn't realize that at any certain point it got—it had deteriorated or had become greater or less so. That's why I am curious to see what you'll say.

Mrs. Wagner: I would say it was worse. (*Mark laughs.*)

Minuchin: Now, why was it worse? Really, at this point, you had a child; you became a mother. How was it? I could understand how it was worse for him; how did it become worse for you?

Mrs. Wagner: He didn't change. He might have needed me, but he never showed that he needed me. He never once said, "I need you," you know. He never once said, "This is great," you know, "being a family," and everything. Ummm. I can't think of my train of thought.

Minuchin: Did you—did you—change towards him, then? When you had Tommy? Did you become—certainly you must have become less available to him.

Mrs. Wagner: Oh, right. I mean. I don't think I changed any. I think I might have—yeah, I think I got progressively worse as far as my attitude toward him was. I felt like, you've got me in this rut and now I'm stuck.

Minuchin: You in effect were stuck and he was unstuck. He could move out; you couldn't. Did you tell him that?

Mrs. Wagner: I told him to go a lot of times; but he didn't want to leave.

Minuchin: At this point, you didn't want him.

Mrs. Wagner: Oh, I felt I—well, let's see—I had had it. But we had our ups and downs, I think. We'd get along horribly for three weeks and then get along all right for one week. This was great, you know, this was the way it was supposed to be like, and then we would go back to the same vicious cycle. But I must point out that in the whole time that we did get along, I mean everybody has their ups and downs, even now, but we never once had an argument over anything of any value, or importance; it was over like who would take out the rubbish; it was never over anything that had anything major to do with our lives.

Minuchin: Who took out the rubbish?

Mrs. Wagner: I'd say, "Mark, take out the rubbish." We had rats, you know.

Minuchin: And?

Mrs. Wagner: "I'll do it when I get around to it."

Mr. Wagner: "Yes, and I'll do it on my own time" (*laughs*).

Mrs. Wagner: In the meantime, it would overflow, and then we would have a big fight, you know. The rubbish was overflowing, just little things like that. It was never over anything important.

Minuchin: You could not accept that that was just a question of the rubbish. You were making it a question of—authority.

Mrs. Wagner: That's right.

Mr. Wagner: I am willing to do what you ask me to do, provided that you don't expect me to do it, you know, as you want me to do it—

Mrs. Wagner: Or on time.

Minuchin: How did the rubbish get transported—

Mr. Wagner: It was just a little thing, and all these things she mentioned were little things—ah—

Minuchin: Life is made up of little things.

Mr. Wagner: That was just my way of showing resistance or—what?

Minuchin: I think that you were saying all the time, "I am single." You know?

Mrs. Wagner: He could have been.

Minuchin: You were saying to him, "You are married. Take out the garbage. That's a married function" (*laughs*). He was saying, "I am single."

Mrs. Wagner: He was not helpful. I mean, he never changed a diaper until Tommy was six months old—and that started right from the beginning. I said, "Mark, you've got to learn how to change the diaper— what if I get sick or something's going to happen. You're going to have to change a diaper." Well, I couldn't go out of the house unless I took the baby with me because the baby might disturb him when he was studying. And so—right there—that brings up a conflict—

Child rearing offers many opportunities for individual growth and for strengthening the family system. At the same time, it is a field in which many fierce battles are fought. Often, unresolved conflicts of the spouses are brought piggyback into the area of child rearing because the couple cannot separate parenting functions from spouse functions.

Minuchin: Let me go out on a limb. I bet Mark's mother is a very efficient person, who did a lot of things for him.

Mr. Wagner: Yes. Yes, in that sense she is. She perhaps is not an efficient housekeeper.

Minuchin: I am talking about the other things.

Mr. Wagner: Right. She was the person you went to to get—

Mrs. Wagner: She did things for you.

Mr. Wagner: If you had a decision that you were having a problem resolving, she was the person that would help you resolve it. Generally speaking, her way was generally right, or appeared to be.

Minuchin: You know—what I am talking about is what kind of expectations did you have of Emily.

Mr. Wagner: Okay. Whereas my mother was always there with whatever we needed—

Mrs. Wagner: I must say, he never—he never told me what he expected of me as a wife. I told him. I used to say what I expected of him as a husband, but he never said, "I expect this of you as a wife." We never sat down and said what we expected of each other, which was wrong right from the start, you know. We never even sat—we just—you know—we just went into this marriage, "Hey, this is going to be fun," you know. We never knew what to expect from one another.

Mr. Wagner: Probably, I had tried to change her and she just said, "Forget it."

Mrs. Wagner: Yeah, he expected certain things of me, like, oh, I'll start out like, when we were dating. I wasn't supposed to smoke in public and I wasn't supposed to bleach my hair and I wasn't supposed to do that—

Minuchin: Is your hair bleached?

Mrs. Wagner: Now it is.

Minuchin: But that means that there has been accommodation.

Mrs. Wagner: An example—we were—we were in Kansas, oh maybe a month, and we were able to live in the College Courts and all the girls had frosted their hair. This was just one small example, so I said, "I'm going to frost my hair," and he said, "All right, you frost your hair, I'm going to get a Yul Brynner." It was just the point, you know; I was defying his wishes and he was going to fight me with—and I said, "You're not fighting with me; you're just going to have to fight with yourself because you're the one that is going to look ridiculous." Something like that would start a battle for five months, you know. I went against his wishes.

Minuchin: You know, this what you are describing is so familiar. It happened to me and it happened to all our people around us. So what happened then? Tommy was growing up, and now you had three people instead of two. Now, you had a model that you learned from your home: that Papa and Mama fight through me. That you described as the model in your home.

Mrs. Wagner: But I never realized that until you just said it.

Minuchin: Okay, but let's—let's bring it now to Tommy and see if this model—

Mrs. Wagner: I'd say we did. Definitely, oh, definitely we used Tommy to fight. I would get mad at Mark and lock him out, and he would stand out there and pound on the door, and I would take Tommy to the window and—this was awful—point to him—and say, "See, Tommy, see the funny man," and we'd stand there and make faces at him.

Mr. Wagner: Yeah (*laughs*).

Mrs. Wagner: He'd be standing there, dying, ready to kill both—kill me because I was instigating that little baby, you know—

Minuchin: You transferred a family model that you learned at your home into your marriage.

Mrs. Wagner: I think I did at first, yes.

Minuchin: How did you break that, because that's a very pernicious kind of thing. How did you break it?

Mr. Wagner: Ah. If you say, really a changing point, we reached a crisis, or critical period when I had said to her, uhhh, "We either see a marriage counselor or you may as well forget the whole thing. I think it would be ridiculous to forget it until we find out at least what our problems are, and if we can't communicate, perhaps a person can help us to communicate. Maybe it isn't as serious as we think it is; perhaps just a lot of little things have built up." So we did see a marriage counselor, about a year ago.

Minuchin: Okay. Now then, you said that the critical point was when, when you left Kansas?

Mrs. Wagner: Ummm hmmm. It was about four or five months after we—

Minuchin: After you came here. Well, but you see a number of changes occurred now. You were not a student any more. This is the first time that you really didn't have a road you could traverse undisturbed. So what happened to you?

Mr. Wagner: Here I am moving into a new position; we've moved locations entirely; it's an entirely different type of life. I, in the back of my mind, rationalized that when we got out of there—got out of this situation—things would improve. But they didn't improve. If anything, they probably became worse.

Minuchin: In what way?

Mr. Wagner: As far as I was concerned, you see, they became worse, because I couldn't control them, the way I could—I felt that I could—in this other atmosphere—this small college—I—

Minuchin: How did you support your family when you were in Kansas?

Mr. Wagner: I had a summer job, so I didn't see her in the summer, either. Even when we—were married.

Minuchin: Did that—that kept you financially?

Mr. Wagner: For the most part. I borrowed money; I worked at school, and did this during the summer.

Minuchin: Did your parents help you or you—?

Mrs. Wagner: My parents did. And his parents did, too.

Minuchin: So, your families are still very much in the picture. Some-times, you know, that makes for difficulties in defining the new marriage.

Mr. Wagner: I would say that they were very much beneficial, though. They gave us something to fall back on.

Minuchin: I am saying that it creates another dimension. What happened when you came here? What did you think you were going to do?

Mr. Wagner: I—well, I had envisioned that once I was working full time—

Minuchin: In what? You graduated—

Mr. Wagner: I graduated with a double major in business and biology.

Minuchin: So you came here. What are you doing?

Mr. Wagner: Working as an office manager in town.

Minuchin: Is that what you trained for?

Mr. Wagner: Yes, generally speaking.

Mrs. Wagner: No.

Minuchin: You said "no" and he said "yes."

Mr. Wagner: Yes, in a general way. Yeah.

Mrs. Wagner: I wouldn't say that he is happiest in it.

Mr. Wagner: Well, number one, my greatest interest is in biology, but it isn't practical for me to make a living at it, because I have no desire to teach, to do research, and I can't afford to go to medical school, so—this is why I picked up the business major in my junior year, realizing that biology would have to be more of an avocation, and picked up business, which was a second choice.

Minuchin: So, now you are working and you are supporting your family. You are supporting your family totally?

Mr. Wagner: No.

Mrs. Wagner: I'm working, too.

Mr. Wagner: She just started to work a short time ago. It's not abso-lutely necessary, but—

Mrs. Wagner: It was by choice; it was my own decision.

Minuchin: So that means this is a big change in your life. Now you are not any more a student, and groups are not any more organized for you.

Mr. Wagner: Not only that, but when I leave work, that's the end of work; I go home; I don't have any studying to do, or anything else, so

I channel that towards the family. If I—if there's no satisfaction in this, I realize I better do something about it, because this is my life, you see, whereas before I could shut it out. Here I have no outlet. Either I live with it, or I do something about it.

Minuchin: So, it seems as if this is the first time in which you really make a commitment.

Mr. Wagner: Ummm hummm. In a sense—

Minuchin: Now you are stuck also.

The changed circumstances of the Wagners' lives are paralleled by changes in the family. Mark is no longer a student. He has moved to a more independent position in the outside world, where he now has autonomy and responsibility. Now there is a clearer demarcation between the family and the extrafamilial. When he comes home, he is home. He no longer brings the extrafamilial tasks home with him.

Complementary changes have occurred for Emily. She has now taken a job, which is giving her a sense of effectiveness, or competence, in the outside world. Less time is devoted to the family, but this makes the time she does spend on being a wife and mother more satisfactory.

Minuchin: You see, up to now, Emily, you were stuck, and he was a student. So you (*to husband*) come here and you make a commitment to the family. And at this point it stinks.

Mr. Wagner: Ummm hummm.

Minuchin: Okay, so then it is that you decide to see—

Mr. Wagner: Yeah, I decided that we had to see a marriage counselor. We did. As it turned out, we only had to see him four times before we both changed radically. And since then we have been getting along very well.

Mrs. Wagner: We still have—you know, arguments—

Mr. Wagner: Oh yes, but still it's not a continuing thing—

Minuchin: You are lucky. Some marriage counselors get hooked into families, and they don't let them go.

Mrs. Wagner: When we went in, I said, "If this can't be saved, we might as well contemplate—" I met this guy—we enjoyed him, you know. He was great. He said, "You basically have a good marriage, if you would both just shut up and start listening to each other and stop working against each other," and—

Minuchin: And just that helped you?

Mr. Wagner: No, it wasn't really that. It was the atmosphere and the fact that he was intelligent enough so that he knew when we weren't telling the truth.

Mrs. Wagner: I didn't tell the truth for about three sessions (*laughs*).

Mr. Wagner: If you didn't tell the truth, well, you looked pretty silly.

Mrs. Wagner: I just sat there, ummm hummm, and he said, "That's not what I want to hear," you know—anything that was bothering me, I kept inside myself and, you know, it was none of anybody's business. And he'd sit there, "Emily, you're not telling me the truth," you know, and he'd really make me dig at my own thoughts and stop and think before I said something.

Minuchin: And what did he do to you?

Mr. Wagner: Well, maybe he realized that I wasn't being entirely truthful with myself, number one. And also, it was the first real opportunity that I had had to listen to what she really was saying.

Minuchin: You know, I would disagree. I think you were truthful to yourself; I think you were not truthful to your marriage. You were, you know, doing your own thing.

If at this point in their marital relationship the focus of exploration had been the individual realities of Mark and Emily instead of the reality of their complementarity, it is possible that the marriage would have broken up.

Mr. Wagner: Ummm hummm, but I didn't—there were a lot of things that I was overlooking as faults within myself, that I perhaps couldn't see subjectively, but objectively—

Mrs. Wagner: I was carrying all this guilt that he was fair and it was all my fault. You know? I had failed and that was it. We've got to call it quits and get it over and done with, and the sooner the better.

Minuchin: And he helped you to work it out.

Mrs. Wagner: Ummm hummm.

Mr. Wagner: Ummm hummm.

Minuchin: Okay, let's stop it here. Are there any questions from the audience?

Question: I had a question about the kinds of things that you were interested in asking these people, the kinds of things you would discuss in this kind of interview, as opposed to a therapy interview, when somebody comes who is hurting about something.

Minuchin: Our colleague was asking before, in private, if there were certain things about this interview that were not stressful enough. I was not picking at areas of stress. I told him that I thought that you were a normal family, and that means that you were as mixed up as he was, like many other families. You went through the routes that many of us traverse. What you went through, it seems to me, is the tremendous amount of difficulties that people have in forming a family. They come from different cultures with different ideas, and they meet, strangers. They need to create boundaries around themselves, and they struggle. And they struggle and they blunder and they have bloody noses, right? All of us have. And you know, some marriages survive, and some don't. But we all go through that, in different ways.

Question: I'm not clear on why there were only four meetings with the marriage counselor, and how it was decided to stop.

Mr. Wagner: You might say that he broke the shell; he broke down the barrier, and then we were able to communicate ourselves, and since we had communicated so candidly during our counseling, you see, there was nothing held back or anything, and we both realized that we both made mistakes.

Question: I gather there was a point in your life in particular when you were ready to offer something—

Mr. Wagner: Where previously I wasn't.

Question: Yeah—you were able to negotiate—

Mr. Wagner: Probably as much timing as anything else.

Question: I have a couple of questions to ask. During the time at first when all that was going on, did you ever leave him?

Mrs. Wagner: Yes. We went on a camping trip, which was a terrible experience. He was taking a field biology course in the middle of the woods, and I was there maybe three weeks, and I was miserable: he was gone all day, and there were no neighbors—I was nine miles from town in the middle of the woods, with nobody around me. It was just terrible to begin with, and nobody but Tommy, and he had classes at night; it was like a lab workshop, really, and he had classes at night, and one day, I just called up home and said, "Please send me the money; I can't stand this," and I went home, and I was only going to stay for a week—I stayed two weeks, and then I came back and we went back to Kansas for a visit and I brought Tommy back with me just so I would have company, you know.

Question: Were you pretty afraid when you left him?

Mrs. Wagner: When I got home, I was very homesick for him. I was afraid, but when I got back, I thought maybe we'll get along good, and I think we did for the first day, and the next day we went right back into our old routine. I felt like it wasn't worth coming back.

Question: I suspect that even when people put up walls, they still communicate in other ways if they keep contact. And I think that this is part of it, you know, really, the sense that comes through today, of your being very much in contact. You do check with each other about a lot of things, as you talk. You may interrupt each other, and you interrupt him more than he does you—

Mrs. Wagner: Oh, definitely—

Question: And so forth, but there's an awful lot of communication that's going on in the way that you look at each other and check with each other about certain things, using your bodies and your eyes, etc., which I think goes on in families, which is a way of communication that we don't usually underscore as we talk about it. That kind of caring may well be there, while you may be mad as hell about the garbage and mad as hell about the rules, there are other things that are going on, and I suspect that these are the things that are both demonstrated in relation to Tommy, and are demonstrated in relation to each other. There isn't a malevolence of anger, the anger really is not any kind of—while it's painful, I didn't catch it as being "out to kill."

Mr. Wagner: It was more—more spurious.

Mrs. Wagner: No, it was more to hurt, more than anything. When I came home when I left, I wasn't mad at him; I was sick, and I just got miserable; I was more lonely than anything, because he wasn't there, or anything. I mean, my mother's phone bill during those two weeks was $40, just for two weeks. We were continuously calling back and forth, you know. It was just that we went back to the same old pattern. It was an unhealthy atmosphere when I left, and I came back to the same atmosphere. Neither of us had changed during those two weeks.

Question: You were mentioning the things that you couldn't rely on each other for, like garbage, and I am wondering what you now, each of you, mainly relies on the other for.

Minuchin: What are the ways in which you support each other?

Mrs. Wagner: Now? I think that—as far as husbands go, I couldn't have a better husband, better provider; he's very helpful; there isn't anything he won't do for me, as far as efficiency—

Mr. Wagner: This was something that we had to work out between the two of us—ah—

Mrs. Wagner: He never would do anything before on his own, but now I can't stop him. He helps me—he's at it constantly. Of course, I think it came when he got more adjusted to marriage; once he was happy, he took enjoyment in making our home nice and everything else, you know.

Mr. Wagner: See, I never had to do these things in college, because you always did them for me, so I didn't do it anyway. I just said, "I'll do it later." Then there was a very good chance you would do it.

The change in the husband's behavior is accompanied by a complementary change in the wife's interaction with him. Or is it the other way around?

Question: There is another thing that is striking and very appealing about this, which Dr. Minuchin pointed out at one point, and it is that, Mrs. Wagner's reaction is like an affective barometer, and usually Mr. Wagner balances this by a very logical interpretation. So there is a kind of vitality that Mrs. Wagner can lend to a logical interpretation, and by the same token, there's a lot of toning down. That's when it works well, but we have seen a lot of people who have the same separation of roles, with one being the one who does the thinking out process, the other does the feeling; they don't seem to work as a team about it . . . So there's another quality. Given that other quality, these two work beautifully, as you have pointed out. It doesn't seem quite as fragmented as I am describing, because I think, they both do everything; in a way, there's more overlap possibly than we think.

Minuchin: Well, for a number of years it did not work. I think that probably one of the things that happened was Mark's lack of commitment to being married, huh? That you kept longer being a single person than she did.

Mr. Wagner: Oh, much longer—that's true. To her I was a know-it-all you see, and when she'd call me a know-it-all, it just went against my nature. I won't even begin to discuss anything. I mean that would end it; that's why we never could get anywhere. I'd say something or suggest something and probably be a little overbearing about it, and she would say, "Well, you're a know-it-all, anyway," and that was the end of it. I had to learn to take a few punches and roll a little bit, and to give in. You'll notice someone commented that she interrupted me more than I interrupted her. Ah—this is just about the opposite of the way it would have been a year or two ago.

Mrs. Wagner: Actually, if we have a normal conversation, Mark will monopolize. I was—I have to interrupt him, usually, in order to get anything in. When he gets going, I really can't get anything in. He still, in that sense, is in his own world. You say something—even that you have the same interest in it as him, but no, you can't get a word in.

Question: I was wondering what, that went on today, had meaning to you two, a different kind of meaning?

Mr. Wagner: Quite a few things. He pointed out something that perhaps isn't really, wouldn't appear to be important. He noticed that in this relationship, I tend to understate. She tends to go in the other direction, and I never really was aware of it, not consciously, at least, that this was the case. I always qualify what she says.

Mrs. Wagner: Protecting me against myself.

Mr. Wagner: I feel that sometimes she puts her foot in her mouth.

Mrs. Wagner: I do.

Mr. Wagner: She goes too far, you see. She just makes a blatant generalization, boom—I come back and say, "Well, yeah, but—" It's my nature to do this, good or bad.

Question: What was the dramatic change as you became committed?

Mr. Wagner: Oh, I don't think it was that dramatic a change—I think, below the surface, it wasn't that bad a relationship. It was just these little things, the stubbornness—these certain things that are always going to be incongruous, always tight against each other on the surface, and this blocked a lot of communication that could have been—but we still had understanding. As you say, it was a different sort of communication.

Mrs. Wagner: We still have days when we hate each other, and it's only normal.

Mr. Wagner: In relation to Tommy, there hasn't been any real change there, I mean, as a go-between that might exist in our marriage. There has been some change as far as our give and take relative to views on child raising, but that was just a result of the general abilities to give and take that we have acquired at this time, and a lot of things have resulted from that.

Question: Can you tell us about those things?

Mr. Wagner: Specifically, I'm perhaps more lax about this in raising Tommy. When a child says "no" to me, I don't shudder. I try to make him understand that, you know, you don't say "no." Her manner of handling is a little different: if you say "no," well, zap, you get it. You don't say "no" to her. There's a little difference of opinion there.

I think probably, though, that her way is as right as mine, but as long as he buys it, then she accepts my way of doing it, and I accept her way of doing. Previously, this was a source of argument; there was no give and take—it was either one way or the other. Now, it's sort of a compromise, between the two. We've adopted each other's methods, at least more so than previously. That's about as much as I can say. Another way of putting it—when two people decide to make a change, it's a bit different when one does and one doesn't. We made an agreement for change. I think she was waiting for a change long before I ever decided that I would effect a change; she was anticipating this change, was waiting for it, in a sense, so that when I decided there would be a change, and applied myself to it, it was easy for her to follow through. If you see what I mean, she had herself geared that way.

3 A Family Model

Man survives in groups; this is inherent in the human condition. An infant's most basic need is for a mother figure to feed, protect, and teach him. Beyond that, man has survived in all societies by belonging to social aggregates. In different cultures these aggregates vary in their level of organization and differentiation. Primitive societies rely on large groupings with a stable distribution of functions. As societies grow more complex and new skills are required, societal structures are differentiated. Modern urban industrial civilization makes two conflicting demands on man: the ability to develop highly specialized skills, and the capacity for rapid adaptation to a constantly changing socioeconomic scene. The family has always undergone changes that parallel society's changes. It has taken over or given up the functions of protecting and socializing its members in response to the culture's needs. In this sense, family functions serve two different ends. One is internal—the psychosocial protection of its members; the other is external—the accommodation to a culture and the transmission of that culture.

Urban industrial society has intruded forcefully on the family, taking over many functions that were once considered the family's duties. The old now live apart, in old people's homes or in housing developments for senior citizens. Economic support is provided by society through social security or welfare. The young are educated by schools, mass media, and peers. The value of what used to be women's

46

work has been drastically curtailed by modern technology, which has changed tasks necessary for the survival of the family unit to drudgery that a machine can do better. Conditions that allow or require both spouses to work outside the family create situations in which the extrafamilial network may heighten and exacerbate conflict between the spouses.

In the face of all these changes, modern man still adheres to a set of values that belong to a different society, one in which the boundaries between the family and the extrafamilial were clearly delineated. The adherence to an outmoded model leads to the labeling of many situations that are clearly transitional as pathological and pathogenic. The touchstone for family life is still the legendary "and so they were married and lived happily ever after." It is no wonder that any family falls short of this ideal.

The occidental world is in a state of transition, and the family, which must always accommodate to society, is changing with it. But because of transitional difficulties, the family's major psychosocial task—to support its members—has become more important than ever. Only the family, society's smallest unit, can change and yet maintain enough continuity to rear children who will not be "strangers in a strange land," who will be rooted firmly enough to grow and to adapt.

THE MATRIX OF IDENTITY

In all cultures, the family imprints its members with selfhood. Human experience of identity has two elements: a sense of belonging and a sense of being separate. The laboratory in which these ingredients are mixed and dispensed is the family, the matrix of identity.

In the early process of socialization, families mold and program the child's behavior and sense of identity. The sense of belonging comes with an accommodation on the child's part to the family groups and with his assumption of transactional patterns in the family structure that are consistent throughout different life events. Tommy Wagner is a Wagner, and throughout his life he will be the son of Emily and Mark. This will be an important facto: in his existence. That Mark is the father of Tom is an important factor in Mark's life, as is the fact that he is the husband of Emily. Every member's sense of identity is influenced by his sense of belonging to a specific family.

The sense of separateness and individuation occurs through participation in different family subsystems in different family contexts, as well as through participation in extrafamilial groups. As the child and the family grow together, the accommodation of the family to the child's needs delimits areas of autonomy that he experiences as separateness. A psychological and transactional territory is carved out for that particular child. Being Tom is different from being a Wagner.

But every individual's sense of identity is influenced by his sense of belonging to different groups. Part of Mark Wagner's identity is the fact that he is the father of Tom and the husband of Emily, as well as the child of his parents. The components of an individual's sense of identity change and remain constant. As Roger Barker put it, "the psychological person who writes essays, scores points, and crosses streets stands as an identifiable entity between unstable interior parts and exterior contexts, with both of which he is linked, yet from both of which he is profoundly separated."[1] The psychological person who is a separate entity is linked with exterior contexts.

Although the family is the matrix of its members' psychosocial development, it must also accommodate to society and ensure some continuity to its culture. This societal function is the source of attacks on the family in modern America. American society is changing, and many groups within that society want to hurry the change. These groups see the family, quite correctly, as an element of conservatism and a source of stasis. Attacks on the family are typical of revolutionary periods. Christ told his disciples to leave their parents and families and to follow him. The French, Russian, and Chinese revolutions all undermined the traditional family structure in those countries in an attempt to speed the progress toward a new social order. The Israeli kibbutz is another example of the same social process.

Russian laws bearing on the family during and after their revolution illustrate this process. In the 1920s, laws regulating marriage, divorce, and abortion tended toward the dissolution of the family. But in the 1930s, when Russia was moving toward the crystallization of its newly established societal norms, laws were changed to support family continuity.[2] Similarly, the Israeli kibbutzim are now tending to increase the functions of the nuclear family within the kibbutz. In many of them, infants now stay in their parents' room, and children live with their parents for a longer time before joining the children's home.

Any study of the family must include its complementarity to

society. The nuclear family, which in theory at least is the American middle class norm, is a recent historical development. Even today, it is largely confined to urban industrialized societies. Concepts of family functions also change as society changes. Up to four hundred years ago, the family was not seen as a child-rearing unit, and not until much later were children recognized as individuals in their own right.[3]

Today the American family, like American society, is in a transitional period. And like the society it transmits, the family is under attack. For example, a twelve-hour public educational television program, "An American Family," followed the Loud family through the routines of their life and their relationships with jobs, schools, in-laws, and friends. Some people hailed this presentation as a breakthrough in mass media communication, with significant anthropological value. Others criticized the dullness of the presentation of family life. One significant critical group was the Loud family itself. On independent television shows they tried to communicate to an audience of millions that they did not like themselves as they were portrayed. They pointed out that there was much more to them than was shown. What the American audience saw was in fact the producer's point of view. Influenced by current views of the family, he had selected and highlighted excerpts that exemplified these views. Similar distortions were made by the cameramen and crew, who framed the shots, selected closeups, and pinpointed what they considered to be the relevant aspects of the family. Americans saw an American family presented according to cultural views of the family that are currently fashionable.

Attacks on the family are coming from many sources. Joining in are the intellectual leaders of the counterculture movement and groups of young people who have been experimenting with communal forms of family organization and child rearing. In the mental health field, R.D. Laing and his followers have been influential in portraying the family as the malevolent programmer of psychosis and, even worse, of the "normal" adults that populate our world.[4] The new feminist movement has also attacked the family, describing it as an entrenchment of male chauvinism. They see the nuclear family as an organization that cannot help but produce little girls reared to be wives in the doll house, and little boys who will be just as trapped in outmoded patterns.

The family will change as society changes. Probably in complementary fashion, society will develop extrafamilial structures to adapt to new currents of thought and new social and economic realities. The 1970s seem to be an interim period of struggle, during which changes are creating a need for structures that have not yet appeared. The large number of families in which both parents work outside the home, for example, has created a need for day care services on a large scale, which are not yet available.

The generation gap is another example of unmet needs. The family is relinquishing the socialization of children earlier and earlier. The school, mass media, and the peer group are taking over the guidance and education of older children. But society has not developed adequate extrafamilial sources of socialization and support.

The Masai society had an adolescent peer group culture that was largely independent but was assigned certain specific tasks for the group to perform under the laissez-faire supervision of the tribe's warriors. The youths could thus carry out the age-appropriate processes of separating from the family and becoming independent without becoming alienated from society at large. The youth groups of the Israeli kibbutzim perform a similar function. Western society does not have clearly differentiated functions for adolescents. When the family releases its children, it releases them to inadequate supporting systems. It is not surprising that adolescent crises of identity have resulted in a number of antinomian social phenomena.[5]

Change always moves from society to the family, never from the smaller unit to the larger. The family will change, but it will also remain, because it is the best human unit for rapidly changing societies. The more flexibility and adaptiveness society requires from its members, the more significant the family will become as the matrix of psychosocial development.

As the family, in a generic sense, changes and adapts to historical circumstances, so the individual family constantly adapts. The family is an open system in transformation; that is, it constantly receives and sends inputs to and from the extrafamilial, and it adapts to the different demands of the developmental stages it faces.

Its tasks are not easy. The Wagners, with all the difficulties they describe in family formation and the birth of their child, typify the stresses that any normal family encounters. But somehow, the prevailing idealized view of the normal family is that it is nonstressful. In spite of sociological and anthropological studies of the family, the myth of placid normality endures, supported by hours of two-dimensional television characters. This picture of people living in harmony, coping with social inputs without getting ruffled, and always cooperating with each other, crumbles whenever one looks at any family with its ordinary problems. It is therefore alarming that this standard is sometimes maintained unchallenged by therapists, who measure the functioning of client families against the idealized image. Freud pointed out that therapy changes neurotic patterns into the normal miseries of life. His comment is just as true for family therapy.

Since a normal family cannot be distinguished from an abnormal family by the absence of problems, a therapist must have a conceptual schema of family functioning to help him analyze a family. A schema based on viewing the family as a system, operating within specific social contexts, has three components. First, the structure of the family is that of an open sociocultural system in transformation. Second, the family undergoes development, moving through a number of stages that require restructuring. Third, the family adapts to changed circumstances so as to maintain continuity and enhance the psychosocial growth of each member. The interview with the Wagners was designed to uncover the second component of this schema, their developmental stages, with the commentary presenting more generic aspects of family development. Family structure and family adaptation require further discussion.

FAMILY STRUCTURE

Family structure is the invisible set of functional demands that organizes the ways in which family members interact. A family is a system that operates through transactional patterns. Repeated transactions establish patterns of how, when, and to whom to relate, and these patterns underpin the system. When a mother tells her child to drink his juice and he obeys, this interaction defines who she is in relation to him and who he is in relation to her, in that context and at that time. Repeated operations in these terms constitute a transactional pattern.

In their interview the Wagners described many such patterns. Emily generally plans the family's Saturday activities, but only an event of major importance would make her interfere with her husband's Sunday fishing trip. In her family of origin, Emily was involved in a coalition with her mother against her father: the mother encouraged the daughter to disobey the father, who complemented this by attacking the daughter when he was angry at the mother.

Transactional patterns regulate family members' behavior. They are maintained by two systems of constraint. The first is generic, involving the universal rules governing family organization. For instance, there must be a power hierarchy, in which parents and children have different levels of authority. There must also be a complementarity of functions, with the husband and wife accepting interdependency and operating as a team.

The second system of constraint is idiosyncratic, involving the mutual expectations of particular family members. The origin of these expectations is buried in years of explicit and implicit negotiations among family members, often around small daily events. Frequently the nature of the original contracts has been forgotten, and they may never have even been explicit. But the patterns remain—on automatic pilot, as it were—as a matter of mutual accommodation and functional effectiveness.

Thus the system maintains itself. It offers resistance to change beyond a certain range, and maintains preferred patterns as long as possible. Alternative patterns are available within the system. But any deviation that goes beyond the system's threshold of tolerance elicits mechanisms which re-establish the accustomed range. When situations of system disequilibrium arise, it is common for family members to feel that other members are not fulfilling their obligations. Calls for family loyalty and guilt-inducing maneuvers then appear.[6]

But the family structure must be able to adapt when circumstances change. The continued existence of the family as a system depends on a sufficient range of patterns, the availability of alternative transactional patterns, and the flexibility to mobilize them when necessary. Since the family must respond to internal and external changes, it must be able to transform itself in ways that meet new circumstances without losing the continuity that provides a frame of reference for its members.

The family system differentiates and carries out its functions through subsystems. Individuals are subsystems within a family. Dyads such as husband-wife or mother-child can be subsystems. Subsystems can be formed by generation, by sex, by interest, or by function.

Each individual belongs to different subsystems, in which he has different levels of power and where he learns differentiated skills. A man can be a son, nephew, older brother, younger brother, husband, father, and so on. In different subsystems, he enters into different complementary relationships. People accommodate kaleidoscopically to attain the mutuality that makes human intercourse possible. The child has to act like a son as his father acts like a father; and when the child does so, he may have to cede the kind of power that he enjoys when interacting with his younger brother. The subsystem organization of a family provides valuable training in the process of maintaining the differentiated "I am" while exercising interpersonal skills at different levels.

Boundaries. The boundaries of a subsystem are the rules defining who participates, and how. For example, the boundary of a parental subsystem is defined when a mother (M) tells her older child, "You aren't your brother's parent. If he is riding his bike in the street, tell me, and I will stop him" (Fig. 2). If the parental subsystem includes a

Fig. 2
$$\frac{M}{\text{children}}\quad\begin{array}{l}\text{(executive subsystem)}\\[4pt]\text{(sibling subsystem)}\end{array}$$

parental child (PC), the boundary is defined by the mother's telling the children, "Until I get back from the store, Annie is in charge" (Fig. 3).

Fig. 3
$$\frac{M \text{ and } PC}{\text{other children}}\quad\begin{array}{l}\text{(executive subsystem)}\\[4pt]\text{(sibling subsystem)}\end{array}$$

The function of boundaries is to protect the differentiation of the system. Every family subsystem has specific functions and makes specific demands on its members; and the development of

---

Key to Figs. 2–48

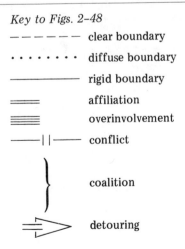

– – – – – –   clear boundary

· · · · · · · ·   diffuse boundary

————   rigid boundary

═══   affiliation

≡≡≡   overinvolvement

——| |——   conflict

}   coalition

⟹   detouring

interpersonal skills achieved in these subsystems is predicated on the subsystem's freedom from interference by other subsystems. For example, the capacity for complementary accommodation between spouses requires freedom from interference by in-laws and children, and sometimes by the extrafamilial. The development of skills for negotiating with peers, learned among siblings, requires noninterference from parents.

For proper family functioning, the boundaries of subsystems must be clear. They must be defined well enough to allow subsystem members to carry out their functions without undue interference, but they must allow contact between the members of the subsystem and others. The composition of subsystems organized around family functions is not nearly as significant as the clarity of subsystem boundaries. A parental subsystem that includes a grandmother or a parental child can function quite well, so long as lines of responsibility and authority are clearly drawn.

The clarity of boundaries within a family is a useful parameter for the evaluation of family functioning. Some families turn upon themselves to develop their own microcosm, with a consequent increase of communication and concern among family members. As a result, distance decreases and boundaries are blurred. The differentiation of the family system diffuses. Such a system may become overloaded and lack the resources necessary to adapt and change under stressful circumstances. Other families develop overly rigid boundaries. Communication across subsystems becomes difficult, and the protective functions of the family are handicapped. These two extremes of boundary functioning are called enmeshment and disengagement. All families can be conceived of as falling somewhere along a continuum whose poles are the two extremes of diffuse boundaries and overly rigid boundaries (Fig. 4). Most families fall within the wide normal range.

Fig. 4

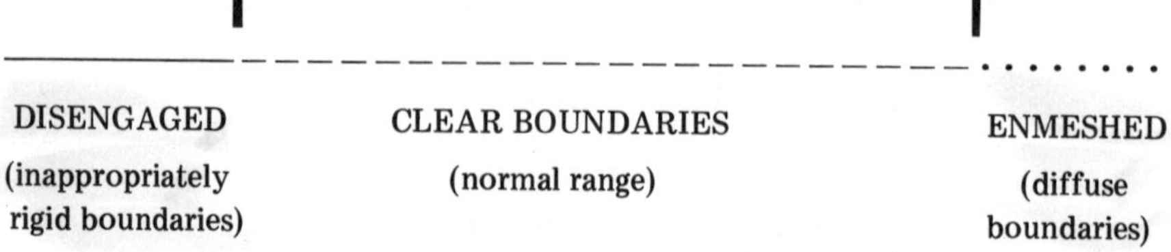

DISENGAGED	CLEAR BOUNDARIES	ENMESHED
(inappropriately rigid boundaries)	(normal range)	(diffuse boundaries)

In human terms, enmeshment and disengagement refer to a transactional style, or preference for a type of interaction, not to a qualitative difference between functional and dysfunctional. Most families have enmeshed and disengaged subsystems. The mother-children subsystem may tend toward enmeshment while the children are small, and the father may take a disengaged position with regard to the children. Mother and younger children can be so enmeshed as to make father peripheral, while father takes a more engaged position with the older children. A parents-child subsystem can tend toward disengagement as the children grow and finally begin to separate from the family.

Operations at the extremes, however, indicate areas of possible pathology. A highly enmeshed subsystem of mother and children, for example, can exclude father, who becomes disengaged in the extreme. The resulting undermining of the children's independence might be an important factor in the development of symptoms.

Members of enmeshed subsystems or families may be handicapped in that the heightened sense of belonging requires a major yielding of autonomy. The lack of subsystem differentiation discourages autonomous exploration and mastery of problems. In children particularly, cognitive-affective skills are thereby inhibited. Members of disengaged subsystems or families may function autonomously but have a skewed sense of independence and lack feelings of loyalty and belonging and the capacity for interdependence and for requesting support when needed.

In other words, a system toward the extreme disengaged end of the continuum tolerates a wide range of individual variations in its members. But stresses in one family member do not cross over its inappropriately rigid boundaries. Only a high level of individual stress can reverberate strongly enough to activate the family's supportive systems. At the enmeshed end of the continuum, the opposite is true. The behavior of one member immediately affects others, and stress in an individual member reverberates strongly across the boundaries and is swiftly echoed in other subsystems.

Both types of relating cause family problems when adaptive mechanisms are evoked. The enmeshed family responds to any variation from the accustomed with excessive speed and intensity. The disengaged family tends not to respond when a response is necessary. The parents in an enmeshed family may become tremendously upset because a child does not eat his dessert. The parents in a disengaged family may feel unconcerned about a child's hatred of school. A therapist often functions as a boundary maker, clarifying diffuse boundaries and opening inappropriately rigid boundaries. His assessment of family subsystems and boundary functioning provides a rapid diagnostic picture of the family, which orients his therapeutic interventions.

The Spouse Subsystem. The spouse subsystem is formed when two adults of the opposite sex join with the express purpose of forming a family. It has specific tasks, or functions, vital to the family's functioning. The main skills required for the implementation of its tasks are complementarity and mutual accommodation. That is, the couple must develop patterns in which each spouse supports the other's functioning in many areas. They must develop patterns of complementarity that allow each spouse to "give in" without feeling he has "given up." Both husband and wife must yield part of their separateness to gain in belonging. The acceptance of mutual interdependence in a symmetrical relationship may be handicapped by the spouses' insistence on their independent rights.

The spouse subsystem can become a refuge from external stresses and the matrix for contact with other social systems. It can foster learning, creativity, and growth. In the process of mutual accommodation, spouses may actualize creative aspects of their partners that were dormant and support the best characteristics of each other. But couples may also activate each other's negative aspects. Spouses may insist on improving or saving their partners, and by this process disqualify them. Instead of accepting them as they are, they impose new standards to be reached. They may establish dependent-protector transactional patterns, in which the dependent member remains dependent so as to protect the partner's feelings of being the protector.

Such negative patterns may exist in average couples without implying an extended pathology or malevolent motivation in either member. If a therapist must challenge a pattern that has become dysfunctional, he should remember to challenge the process without attacking the participants' motivation. A systems-oriented therapist should offer interpretations that underline mutuality, such as, "You protect your wife in a way that inhibits her, and you elicit unnecessary protection from your husband with great skill." A tandem interpretation of this sort emphasizes the complementarity of the system, joins positive and negative in each spouse, and eliminates judgmental implications of motivation.

The spouse subsystem must achieve a boundary that protects it from interference by the demands and needs of other systems. This is particularly true when a family has children. The adults must have a psychosocial territory of their own—a haven in which they can give each other emotional support. If the boundary around the spouses is inappropriately rigid, the system can be stressed by their isolation. But if the spouses maintain loose boundaries, other subgroups, including children and in-laws, may intrude into their subsystem functioning.

In simple human terms, husband and wife need each other as a refuge from the multiple demands of life. In therapy, this need dictates that the therapist protect the boundaries around the spouse subsystem. If the children in a family session interfere with a spouse subsystem transaction, their interference should be blocked. Husband and wife may have sessions that exclude others. If in these sessions they continue to discuss parenting instead of husband-wife transactions, the therapist would do well to point out that they are crossing a boundary.

The Parental Subsystem. A new level of family formation is reached with the birth of the first child. The spouse subsystem in an intact family must now differentiate to perform the tasks of socializing a child without losing the mutual support that should characterize the spouse subsystem. A boundary must be drawn which allows the child access to both parents while excluding him from spouse functions. Some couples who do well as a group of two are never able to make a satisfactory transition to the interactions of a group of three. In some families, the child may be drawn into problems of the spouse subsystem, as happened to Emily Wagner.

As the child grows, his developmental demands for both autonomy and guidance impose demands on the parental subsystem, which must be modified to meet them. The child comes in contact with extrafamilial peers, the school, and other socializing forces outside the family. The parental subsystem must adapt to the new factors impinging on the tasks of socialization. If the child is severely stressed by his extrafamilial environment, that can affect not only his relationship with his parents but even the internal transactions of the spouse subsystem.

The unquestioned authority that once characterized the patriarchal model of the parental subsystem has faded, to be replaced by a concept of flexible, rational authority. Parents are expected to understand children's developmental needs and to explain the rules they impose. Parenting is an extremely difficult process. No one performs it to his entire satisfaction, and no one goes through the process unscathed. Probably it was always more or less impossible. In today's complex, fast-developing society, in which generational gaps occur at smaller and smaller intervals, parenting difficulties have increased.

The parenting process differs depending on the children's age. When children are very young, nurturing functions predominate. Control and guidance assume more importance later. As the child matures, especially during adolescence, the demands made by parents begin to conflict with the children's demands for age-appropriate autonomy. Parenting becomes a difficult process of mutual accommodation. Parents impose rules that they cannot explain at the time or that they explain inadequately, or they regard the reasons for rules as self-evident, when they are not self-evident to the children. As children grow older, they may not accept the rules. The children communicate their needs with varying degress of clarity, and they make new demands on the parents, such as for more time or more emotional commitment.

It is essential to understand the complexity of child rearing in order to judge its participants fairly. Parents cannot protect and guide without at the same time controlling and restricting. Children cannot grow and become individuated without rejecting and attacking. The process of socialization is inherently conflictual. Any therapeutic input that challenges a dysfunctional process between parents and children must at the same time support its participants.

Parenting requires the capacity to nurture, guide, and control. The proportions of these elements depend on the children's developmental needs and the parents' capacity. But parenting always requires the use of authority. Parents cannot carry out their executive functions unless they have the power to do so.

Children and parents, and sometimes therapists, frequently describe the ideal family as a democracy. But they mistakenly assume that a democratic society is leaderless, or that a family is a society of peers. Effective functioning requires that parents and children accept the fact that the differentiated use of authority is a necessary ingredient for the parental subsystem. This becomes a social training lab for the children, who need to know how to negotiate in situations of unequal power.

A therapist's support of the parental subsystem may conflict with a therapeutic goal of supporting a child's autonomy. In such situations, the therapist should remember that only a weak parental subsystem establishes restrictive control, and that excessive control occurs mostly when the control is ineffective. Supporting the parents' responsibility and obligation to determine family rules secures the child's right and obligation to grow and to develop autonomy. The therapist's task is to help the subsystems negotiate with and accommodate to each other.

The Sibling Subsystem. The sibling subsystem is the first social laboratory in which children can experiment with peer relationships. Within this context, children support, isolate, scapegoat, and learn from each other. In the sibling world, children learn how to negotiate, cooperate, and compete. They learn how to make friends and allies, how to save face while submitting, and how to achieve recognition of their skills. They may take different positions in their jockeying with one another, and those positions, taken early in the sibling subgroup, can be significant in the subsequent course of their lives. In large families, the sibling subsystem has a further division, for the younger children, who are still transacting in areas of security, nurturance, and guidance within the family, are differentiated from the older children, who are making contact and contracts with the extrafamilial world.

When children contact the world of extrafamilial peers, they try to operate along the lines of the sibling world. When they learn alternative ways of relating, they bring back the new experiential knowledge into the sibling world. If the child's family has very idiosyncratic ways, the boundaries between the family and the extrafamilial world may become inappropriately rigid. The child may then have difficulty entering other social systems.

The significance of the sibling subsystem is seen most clearly in its absence. Only children develop an early pattern of accommodation to the adult world, which may be manifested in precocious development. At the same time, they may manifest difficulty in the development of autonomy and the ability to share, cooperate, and compete with others.

A therapist should know the developmental needs of children and be able to support the child's right to autonomy without minimizing the parents' rights. The boundaries of the sibling subsystem should protect the children from adult interference, so they can exercise their right to privacy, have their own areas of interest, and be free to fumble as they explore. Children at different developmental stages have different needs, particular cognitive skills, and idiosyncratic value systems. At times, the therapist must act as a translator, interpreting the children's world to the parents or vice versa. He may also have to help the subsystem negotiate clear but crossable boundaries with the extrafamilial. If the child is caught in a web of exaggerated family loyalty, for example, the therapist will act as a bridge between the child and the extrafamilial world.

FAMILY ADAPTATION

A family is subject to inner pressure coming from developmental changes in its own members and subsystems and to outer pressure coming from demands to accommodate to the significant social institutions that have an impact on family members. Responding to these demands from both within and without requires a constant transformation of the position of family members in relation to one another, so they can grow while the family system maintains continuity.

Inherent in this process of change and continuity are the stresses of accommodating to new situations. Family practitioners, in their concentration on family dynamics, may minimize this process, in the same way that dynamic therapists may minimize the context of the individual. The danger of this pitfall is its emphasis on pathology. Transitional processes of adaptation to new situations, which carry the lack of differentiation and the anxiety that characterize all new processes, may be mislabeled as pathological. To focus on the family as a social system in transformation, however, highlights the transitional nature of certain family processes. It demands an exploration of the changing situation of the family and its members and of their stresses of accommodation. With this orientation, many more families who enter therapy would be seen and treated as average families in transitional situations, suffering the pains of accommodation to new circumstances. The label of pathology would be reserved for families who in the face of stress increase the rigidity of their transactional patterns and boundaries, and avoid or resist any exploration of alternatives. In average families, the therapist relies on the motivation of family resources as a pathway to transformation. In pathological families, the therapist needs to become an actor in the family drama, entering into transitional coalitions in order to skew the system and develop a different level of homeostasis.

Stress on a family system may come from four sources. There can be the stressful contact of one member or of the whole family with extrafamilial forces. Transitional points in the family's evolution may also be a source of strain, as are idiosyncratic problems.

Stressful Contact of One Member with Extrafamilial Forces. One of the main functions of the family is to support its members. When a member is stressed, the other family members feel the need to accommodate to his changed circumstances. This accommodation may be contained within a subsystem, or it may permeate the whole family.

For example, a husband, who is under stress at work, criticizes his wife when they both get home. This transaction may be limited to the spouse system. The wife may withdraw from the husband but support him a few minutes later. Or she may counterattack. A fight ensues, but the fight ends with closure and mutual support. These are functional transactional patterns. The stress on the husband has been lessened by the transactions with his wife.

However, the fight may escalate without closure, until one of the spouses abandons the field. Each spouse now suffers from the sense of nonresolution. In this situation, the stressful contact of one family member with external forces has generated an unresolved stress in the intrafamilial spouse subsystem.

The same source of stress on an individual member may operate across subsystem boundaries. For example, a father (F) and mother (M), stressed at work, may come home and criticize each other but then detour their conflict by attacking a child. This reduces the danger to the spouse subsystem, but stresses the child (C) (Fig. 5). Or the

Fig. 5

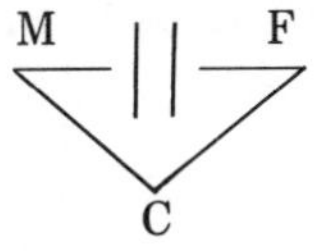

husband may criticize the wife, who then seeks a coalition with the child against the father (Fig. 6). The boundary around the spouse

Fig. 6

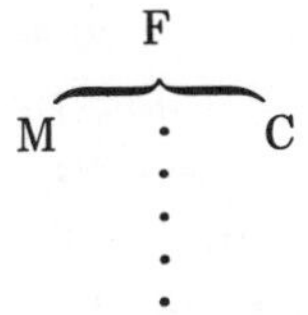

subsystem thereby becomes diffuse. An inappropriately rigid cross-generational subsystem of mother and son versus father appears, and the boundary around this coalition of mother and son excludes the father. A cross-generational dysfunctional transactional pattern has developed.

It is also possible for an entire family to be stressed by one member's extrafamilial contact. For example, if the husband loses his job, the family may have to realign in order to ensure the survival of the family. The wife may have to take on more responsibility for the financial support of the family, thereby changing the nature of the executive subsystem. This change may force changes in the parenting subsystem. The father may take on nurturing functions that were formerly the mother's (Fig. 7). Or a grandmother (G) may be brought

Fig. 7
$$
\begin{array}{ccc}
\text{F} & & \text{M} \\
\underline{\text{M}} & \text{becomes} & \underline{\text{F}} \\
\text{children} & & \text{children}
\end{array}
$$

in to take over parenting functions while both parents are job hunting (Fig. 8). If the family responds to the father's loss of his job with

Fig. 8
$$
\begin{array}{ccc}
\underline{\text{G}} & & \text{M} \\
\text{F} & \text{becomes} & \underline{\text{F}} \\
\underline{\text{M}} & & \underline{\text{G}} \\
\text{children} & & \text{children}
\end{array}
$$

rigidity, dysfunctional transactional patterns may appear. For example, grandmother is brought in to care for the children, but the parents refuse to cede the authority that would enable her to fulfill her responsibility.

The Wagners reported on some of the stresses of contact with the extrafamilial. Mark's difficulties as a student breadwinner interfered with his ability to relate to his wife. He became critical or withdrawn, and Emily brought Tommy into their endless quarrels as her support.

When a family enters therapy because of one member's stressful contact with the extrafamilial, the family therapist's goals and interventions are oriented by his assessment of the situation and of the flexibility of the family structure. If the family has made adaptive changes to support the stressed member but the problem continues, the therapist's main input may be directed toward the interaction of that member with the stressing agent. If the family has not been able to make adaptive changes, his main input may be directed toward the family.

For example, if a child is having trouble in school, the problem may be related basically to the school. If the therapist's assessment indicates that the family is supporting the child adequately, his major interventions will be directed toward the child in the school context. He may act as the child's advocate, arrange a transfer, or arrange for tutoring. But if the child's problems in school seem to be an expression of family problems, the therapist's major interventions will be directed toward the family. Both types of intervention may often be necessary.

Stressful Contact of the Whole Family with Extrafamilial Forces. A family system may be overloaded by the effects of an economic depression. Or stress may be generated by a relocation caused by transfer or urban renewal. Family coping mechanisms are particularly threatened by poverty and discrimination. For example, a poor family may be in contact with so many societal agencies that its coping mechanisms become overloaded. Or a Puerto Rican family may have problems adapting to mainland culture.

Here again, a therapist's interventions will be oriented by his assessment of the family. If he analyzes the family organization and determines that it is basically viable but is overloaded by the impingement of many uncoordinated agencies, he may act as the family's ombudsman. He may teach the family how to manipulate the institutions for its own benefit. Or he may work to coordinate the efforts of the agencies vis-à-vis the family. With a Puerto Rican family overwhelmed by relocation, the family therapist would do well to locate Puerto Rican resources in the community—the church, schools with a large Puerto Rican enrollment, Puerto Rican parents active in the PTA, or social and civic agencies dedicated to helping this ethnic group. His functions as a family therapist will be complemented by his actions as a social matchmaker.

Stress at Transitional Points in the Family. There are many phases in a family's own natural evolution that require the negotiation of new family rules. New subsystems must appear, and new lines of differentiation must be drawn. In this process, conflicts inevitably arise. Ideally, the conflicts will be resolved by negotiations of transition, and the family will adapt successfully. These conflicts offer an opportunity for growth by all family members. However, if such conflicts are not resolved, the transitional problems may give rise to further problems.

Problems of transition occur in a number of situations. They may be produced by developmental changes in family members and by changes in family composition. One of the most common precipitators is the emergence of a child into adolescence. At that time the child's participation in the extrafamilial world and his status in that world increase. The relationship between child and parents is dislocated. The adolescent should be moved a little away from the sibling subsystem and given increased autonomy and responsibility appropriate to his age. The parental subsystem's transactions with him should change from parents-child to parents-young adult. The result will be a successful adaptation (Fig. 9).

Fig. 9

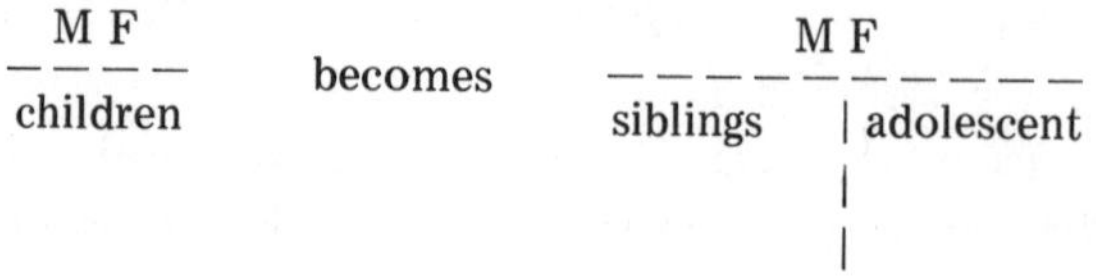

M F
────
children   becomes

M F
────────────
siblings | adolescent
          |
          |

However, the mother may resist any change in her relationship with the adolescent because it would require a change in her relationship with her husband. She may attack the adolescent and undermine his autonomy, instead of changing her own attitude. If the father then enters the conflict on the child's side, an inappropriate cross-generational coalition is formed (Fig. 10). The situation may

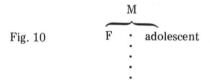

Fig. 10

generalize until the whole family is involved in the conflict. If there is no family change, dysfunctional sets will appear, to be repeated every time a conflict occurs.

When a family absorbs a new member, that new member must adapt to the system's rules, and the old system must be modified to include the new member. There is a tendency to maintain the old patterns, which places a stress on the new member and may cause him to increase his demands. The kinds of increased membership that may produce stress during the period of adaptation are the birth of a child, the marriage of a member of an extended family, the merging of two families through the marriage of single parents, or the inclusion of a relative, friend, or foster child.

Stresses are also produced by adaptation to a decreased membership in a family, caused by such circumstances as the death of a family member, separation or divorce, imprisonment, institutionalization, or a child's leaving for school. For example, when a couple separates, new subsystems and lines of differentiation must develop. The unit of two parents and children must now become a unit of one parent and children, with the other parent excluded.

Families often go into therapy because the negotiations leading to a successful transition have been blocked. A family having problems around a recent transition is easier to help than a family that has blocked adaptive negotiations over a long period.

Stresses Around Idiosyncratic Problems. A family therapist must take all circumstances into account and be aware of the possibility of dysfunctional transactional patterns appearing around idiosyncratic areas of family stress. For example, a family with a retarded child may have been able to adapt to the problems posed while the child was young. But the reality of retardation, which the parents were able to avoid while the child was young, must be faced as he grows older and the disparity of development between the child and his peers becomes more evident.

The same increase of stress may occur when a child with a physical handicap, such as a harelip, grows older. The family may have been able to adapt to the child's needs while he was young, but as the child grows and experiences difficulties in interacting with an extrafamilial peer group that does not accept him, this stress may overload the family system.

Transitory idiosyncratic problems may also overload coping mechanisms. If a family member becomes seriously ill, some of his functions and power must be allocated to other family members. This redistribution requires adaptation in the family. When the sick member recovers, a readaptation to include him in his old position or to help him take a new position in the system becomes necessary.

In summary, the conceptual scheme of a normal family has three facets. First, a family is transformed over time, adapting and restructuring itself so as to continue functioning. A family that has been functioning effectively may nevertheless respond to developmental stresses by adhering inappropriately to previous structural schemas.

Second, the family has a structure, which can be seen only in movement. Certain patterns are preferred, which suffice in response to ordinary demands. But the strength of the system depends on its ability to mobilize alternative transactional patterns when internal or external conditions of the family demand its restructuring. The boundaries of the subsystems must be firm, yet flexible enough to allow realignment when circumstances change.

Finally, a family adapts to stress in a way that maintains family continuity while making restructuring possible. If a family responds to stress with rigidity, dysfunctional patterns occur. These may eventually bring the family into therapy.

4 A Kibbutz Family: The Rabins and Mordecai Kaffman

Esther and Michael Rabin were born in Israel at neighboring kibbutzim and met each other while they were both studying at the regional high school. Up to the age of twelve or thirteen, children study at elementary classes in the kibbutz where they were born and where their parents live. The transfer to a regional high school, called in Hebrew a "Mossad Chinuchi," where youngsters from a number of neighboring kibbutzim study, is an important step in the gradual process of granting independence to the kibbutz younger generation. These schools for adolescents lie near the kibbutzim of the region but not inside them. Like the children's houses for the younger ages, the Mossad is a complete, autonomous unit, providing all the necessary services to its students. They not only study at the Mossad but have a kitchen, dining-room, bedrooms, and clothing services. The frequency of visits by the Mossad students to their parents depends on a number of factors, such as geographical distance, the tradition and custom of the kibbutzim of the specific region, the scholastic load and chores for which the student is responsible, and last but not least, the youngster's own free will. The present trend is for strengthening the contact and increasing the number of visits by the Mossad students to the kibbutzim where their parents live.

Michael is twenty-seven years old and Esther is twenty-six; their only son is nearing three. The young people have known each other since they both joined the same Mossad. The formal wedding took place in 1967. The parents on both sides live in different kibbutzim and belong to the first generation of the founders of their respective kibbutzim.

Kaffman: First, I want to thank you for coming. I have been asked to interview a normal and ordinary family of kibbutz members, so as to find out how this family was formed, to hear how it met, how it acts and gets along, etc. We are interested in knowing how you came to be attached to each other and in what way you approach the common matters of family life. I hope you will talk freely and spontaneously between yourselves or to me. I shall also feel free to talk and interrupt your conversation. The main thing is for everyone to feel free to express whatever he thinks and feels. I wonder what you think about this whole matter?

Mrs. Rabin: Perhaps you will ask questions and then it will be easier.

Kaffman: I have no specific questions. After all, I don't know you. I would simply like to know how you would describe your family life.

Mrs. Rabin: I would prefer Michael to start talking. Otherwise . . .

Kaffman: Ah, it's a hint that he likes to listen a lot and say a little.

Mrs. Rabin: Well, we'd better start. First of all, I don't think that our case is an example of an ordinary couple meeting by accident. We are from the same Mossad; since the eighth class we studied in the same class and since the tenth class, we've been together.

Kaffman: What age was that?

Mrs. Rabin: He was 16½ and I was 15½.

Kaffman: So actually you've got a lot of experience.

Mrs. Rabin: Sure, we're an old family. According to the wedding date, we've been a couple for four years, but in fact a relationship of friendship and love developed between us almost 10 years ago.

Kaffman: So what is unusual about it?

Mrs. Rabin: There was not a situation of a chance meeting or anything sudden; we went around together for quite some time and it wasn't from one day to the next. I think that from the minute it started until the moment it was clear to us that we are a couple, it took about half a year—I mean, until we reached the point of going around together, spending our time together.

Kaffman: In other words, if I understand you correctly, you reached the common feeling that you fitted each other as a couple about half a year after you got to know each other.

Mr. Rabin: It went slowly. I don't think that after half a year we knew we were going to be a couple.

Mrs. Rabin: It was around the end of the tenth class—oh, I get mixed up with the dates—somewhere around Passover that it was said clearly between us that we are attached. Later there were three more years in which we lived together within the same framework the whole day together. In fact, it was worse than family life.

Kaffman: So you say it's not so simple to live too much together.

Mrs. Rabin: It's really not so simple. There are many problems about the relation between the solitary couple and society, and we didn't have the same status in the class, and this period is very critical to the future of the relationship.

Kaffman: I see you are smiling, Michael.

Mr. Rabin: Today we smile at problems that at the time seemed very serious; for example, when we had to take up a stand about social affairs inside the group. It wasn't simple when we had opposite opinions and it wasn't simple when our opinions were uniform. It's difficult to be the first and only couple within such a small framework.

Mrs. Rabin: I think that's right. We never got down to analyzing the situation, but I think that is right. Our situation in class was like this: I was better in studies, but socially my place wasn't so firm, compared to Michael's. You don't think so?

Mr. Rabin: Yes, quite.

Mrs. Rabin: And then, just because of it, a good balance emerged. In anything to do with the social sphere, he held us firmly, and in the area of study, I helped more. Here there were some problems, because our relations were built and destroyed from time to time in this field of studies.

Kaffman: How?

Mrs. Rabin: Well, more than once we used to say, "Business before pleasure," and we had to sit down like good kids to do our homework first, before finding the time for our private affairs. Sometimes it was quite oppressive.

Kaffman: Oppressive in what way? Did you both decide together, or was there a conflict between you about this matter of business before pleasure?

Mrs. Rabin: Many times we both knew in our minds that we had to sit down and study, but our wills weren't so ready for it. But if we finally restrained ourselves and sat down to study, then I, as the better student, had to help him. Well, sometimes you just don't feel like it, and then this sitting together ended up in irritation. Anyway, my attitude then was that I waited impatiently for the moment when we should stop studying, when we should finish high school, so that this factor of studies and the study meetings would not be part of our attachment. Today, each has his own field of study, his own interests, and then there is a much better balance. Now it's not a state where one needs the other's help on unequal terms. In married life there are problems of one sort or another, and each helps the other as best he can. But in an obligation to do your homework, it was not pleasant.

Mr. Rabin: I'll give you another example of the difficulties facing the couple within the group. In the youth movement, there used to be talks, and sometimes a number of members claimed that we two withdrew into ourselves too much and therefore we drifted apart from the collective. So this was one of the problems we had to face and overcome—to bring ourselves back into the collective, as it were. I think that it was very exaggerated, but the social pressure is very strong and you must prove they are wrong. These pressures affect both partners and make it difficult for them.

Kaffman: It sounds as if you were good kids after all. Society wanted you to study more—so you gave up your own personal pleasures. Society wanted you to contribute more actively and be less withdrawn as a couple, so you accepted it after some worrying about it.

Mrs. Rabin: I can't say that we always accepted the pressure of society (*pauses*). As we both were from the same class, the same group, we lived a double life. Suddenly we were one unit of the same class, and we suddenly took ourselves outside the group. Nobody thought anything about a boy taking out his girl when she was from another class. Then everyone knows that at a certain hour she disappears and goes with her boyfriend. But because we were both from the same social unit, our disappearance made itself felt—people realized that the two of us took ourselves outside the group.

Mr. Rabin: Sometimes there is an impression that this friendship is not wanted in the groups at the Mossad. Not always, but sometimes you do feel it. Perhaps this explains the fact that couples within the same group are rare. Maybe they are even jealous of the couple.

Kaffman: And yet you managed to continue for many years under these hard conditions. What actually drew you together?

Mrs. Rabin: I think we are a classic example of what is sometimes called the attraction of opposites. I don't think that there are many couples who are so completely contrasted.

Kaffman: Really, then, this will provide a lot of material on the way you treat the problem of contrast.

Mrs. Rabin: We are very different . . . No, first you, Michael.

Kaffman: You are afraid of influencing him?

Mrs. Rabin: No, I'm afraid that after my words there will be nothing left for him to say.

Mr. Rabin: Analyzing the characters of the two of us is rather complicated. I see myself as a much more calm person. I think this is also expressed in social activities. I get along easily with most people at the kibbutz, without any problems. During my studies I did not achieve very much, but in all youth movement assignments, other activity in the Mossad, various jobs at the kibbutz, there were no problems at all. I was active and cooperated in any social task I was asked to help.

Mrs. Rabin: You don't usually praise yourself; at least do it now. Why don't you go on?

Mr. Rabin: I think it's your turn now.

Kaffman: Earlier you spoke of contrasts. Is everything Michael said about himself different from your character?

Mrs. Rabin: No, no, the main problem, the main difference—I can't express myself in a nutshell—are the quiet, the calmness, the stability which are his main traits, but which don't exist in me. With me everything stands on strain, sometimes negative and sometimes positive, but never an equilibrium. Life for me never flows quietly. And this is why there is much more friction in my relationship with persons. I don't give up. He is much more lenient—towards me too—and I am not. I don't forgive; I get angry very easily. This is how it was, I think, even when I was a young girl. At the Mossad the teachers always used to tell me they don't need an advocate. I have a sort of feeling that my sense of justice is too strong. Every person has it, but many people say, "Why speak, why interfere," and I must react every time. Whatever I think, I say. It's true that many times saying comes before thinking. I think that Michael is different. He is at peace with himself because he knows: "I've done my duty by myself and by others, so it's all right." More than once it happened that someone for whom Michael had done a lot doesn't try to be the same in return, although it's his duty to do so. I feel very deeply hurt, because I tell him, "You did a lot, why should someone else not treat you in the same way?"

Mr. Rabin: But I tell Esther, "Look, let's forget it." And she is more impulsive and was ready to go to war at once.

Mrs. Rabin: That's right, I go to war; with me there is no nonsense. But apparently you are right. You live more quietly, have a better life.

Mr. Rabin: On the whole, these are very small things, not problems of principle. There's no need to flare up so quickly.

Mrs. Rabin: I quite agree that it's right, but still the character remains. And just as I react too sharply to these little things which perhaps don't deserve a reaction, so I sometimes think that he doesn't always react when he should.

Kaffman: Let's hear what happens when you really get hurt.

Mrs. Rabin: He doesn't react either.

Mr. Rabin: Sometimes I say something, but perhaps not firmly enough so that it doesn't happen again. In many cases I really don't react, just swallow it somehow, but in some cases, I do react. I say, you can't always settle every dispute, but even my mild reaction has some effect, I think.

Mrs. Rabin: At this point I have something to add, and here again it's one of the differences. I think that during all the time I have known Michael, I've never seen him insult a person. Such a thing simply doesn't exist for him. Anger, yes, but inside him, quietly, with laughter or with scorn. He gets hurt but does not hurt. I, on the other hand, am quick to hurt and to get hurt. I admit that I can insult people. Sometimes I try to stop myself, but my control is much weaker. Michael is much more balanced. People don't like someone who hurts and gets hurt. It makes them uncomfortable. Now with a person like Michael, who takes his hurt quietly, says nothing, it's much easier.

Kaffman: I wonder whether it is the same in the relationship between you.

Mrs. Rabin: Yes, I admit it is. I'll tell you, there is a joke between us which lasts throughout our life together. I always say that we never quarrel, I simply quarrel with myself. I start a quarrel—Michael doesn't answer. I get more and more angry and irritated. I talk to him, but he keeps quiet and doesn't reply. So, finally, I get reconciled with myself—with him too, but quarreling between us is terribly one-sided, because usually—

Mr. Rabin: I see no reason to turn petty things and passing words into a real quarrel.

Mrs. Rabin: Yes, these are the little things of everyday life when you live in the same room. These quarrels start with me, develop inside me, and finish with me. He takes no part in the quarrels. He just sits quietly and waits, because he knows the storm will pass and everything will come back to normal.

Mr. Rabin: When you are really angry, it's very difficult to put in a word (*laughs*). The trouble is that Esther flares up too quickly, and you must give her some time to cool down a little. Then the problems can be settled much more logically and thoroughly.

Mrs. Rabin: But then these problems don't seem important. Mostly they are really small things. Let's take as an example Michael's help in household chores, keeping the flat clean and neat. I think I don't get enough help from him. So first and last, the quarrel is small and petty, but we have to live here our lives every day and we have to keep the room in order, and give some thought to that. So after all, this small matter becomes important, because it will be with me for all my life, it's not a small matter. It's silly to quarrel about, "Did you or did you not put the kettle on?" and yet it's not silly.

Kaffman: Well, here I see that in fact Michael expresses his objection by failing to do some things in his own quiet way.

Mrs. Rabin: Right. His disagreement is usually expressed in inaction. From time to time, there is a blowup, and then in his own quiet way, Michael gets his say, but things go back to normal, life goes on, and that's it.

Kaffman: I see that Michael still manages in his way to make you angry. When Esther asks for more help with the daily household chores, you don't respond, although just a few minutes ago you described yourself as helping, cooperating, meeting people halfway. Maybe there's no contradiction here. Maybe this inaction has other roots as well. What do you think?

Mr. Rabin: It's true what she says that in many cases I don't do enough, or not at all, such as household chores. But I must say that I really have a very busy working day. For example, I get up at a quarter to six in the morning and can have some rest only at half past eight in the evening.

Kaffman: And until the evening you've no rest?

Mr. Rabin: Yes. So this situation can certainly affect my readiness to do the room, to move the furniture around, to fill the barrel with oil. When I'm too tired, I just don't do it, and this causes friction.

Mrs. Rabin: I understand your reasons, but it's hard to accept. Once again, reason says you are right: after all, when a person gets up early in the morning and doesn't see his bed until 12 at night, it's obvious he doesn't have too much energy left for doing things around the house. With me, the working hours and the whole tempo of the work are not so strenuous.

Kaffman: What work?

Mrs. Rabin: I'm divided: I partly help the doctor at the clinic, and the rest of the time I work at the children's quarters, wherever it's necessary. So however hard I work, and however I believe my day is busy, I always have an hour of rest in the afternoon, before the family time. In the meantime your lord and master comes, he's had no rest today, leave him alone. It really seems like it. It's still hard to accept.

Kaffman: So how do you solve such a problem?

Mrs. Rabin: For example, he works at the factory—there is a workshop there and he could do things I want, a table or a chair. But this is possible only after working hours, and to this I don't agree. So on the one hand, I ask, "Do this and that for me," and on the other hand, "Don't come home late." There's another problem too. I have no hobby and nothing special to do. With him, it's different. Michael has all sorts of hobbies, which take up a lot of his time, and he can't manage them all, so he ends up the loser and he cannot do the things he would have liked to do.

Mr. Rabin: And apart from all that, there are tasks to be done for the kibbutz. As it happened, last year Esther was responsible for the job assignment and I had some other special assignment. And with all this—last and best—we have a little boy.

Mrs. Rabin: At first, it was difficult. It was very difficult to do my job and relax at the hours devoted to spend with the child and taking care of him, especially in periods when Michael had to do his reserve duty in the army. But I think it was a very lovely period just the same.

Kaffman: Was?

Mrs. Rabin: Yes, the good part still continues, but now the burden is not so heavy, because we have finished some of our tasks and now it's much easier.

Kaffman: And you say you are aware of the contradiction between the urge to attack Michael when you feel frustrated and the common sense which Michael represents and which brings you back to reality.

Mrs. Rabin: Yes, and that is why the quarrels are not serious. Anyway, we have no serious problems, as far as I can tell.

Kaffman: So when there is a dispute between you, one of the rules by which the family functions is that Esther flares up, makes some loud criticism, you are able to listen quietly and swallow it all, and then the storm passes. Is that it?

Mrs. Rabin: Just one correction—and it is very important, especially at the kibbutz. Usually, the criticism is not so loud. I do not think the neighbors know about the quarrel. Perhaps they see a sour face or hear some biting remark, but they do not witness any quarrel. It is not done with shouts but usually very quietly. Just a quiet storm. I think it is very good that the neighbors are not part of our private affairs.

Kaffman: So the circle turns round and round in the same direction. How does it affect you?

Mr. Rabin: The truth is that many times I make plans how I would like to surprise Esther by making some new piece of furniture, or doing something around the house, but objectively it is difficult for me to manage it due to this pressure of not enough time. I think this is the problem. It takes time to do what Esther asks me to do. One day we decide to go to Kibbutz Ma'agal to visit my parents. Another time we go to Kibbutz Ganim, where Esther's elder sister lives. It all takes time, of which we do not have too much.

Kaffman: So, you are a rather busy and divided family—rather different from the idyllic picture of the kibbutz which quite a few people have.

Mr. Rabin: Right. With us, it is always "a busy season." There is work, family, the boy, relatives; then one day we go to a play, another day some social work for the kibbutz, and another time there is basketball. So, staying on after work with all this pressure and doing something is—

Mrs. Rabin: And the one evening a week left, you must sleep too (*laughs*).

Kaffman: So, when you do not quarrel, both of you agree that it is just a matter of objective circumstances.

Mr. Rabin: And still, Esther sometimes claims that I am an idler, and there is something in it. I think it is a positive quality.

Mrs. Rabin: A positive quality?

Mr. Rabin (laughs): Yes, in some cases, it is better not to be too diligent.

Mrs. Rabin: Ah, now you have a theory, an ideological basis. If you have principles, I see it is no use nagging you to become more active.

Kaffman: But one thing is certain, as far as I have seen so far. Esther's constant nagging does not in fact activate you.

Mr. and Mrs. Rabin (together): No, it does not.

Kaffman: The question arises in what way this constant nagging does affect you. As it does not rouse you to doing things, perhaps to a certain extent it irritates you and causes your inactivity. Perhaps here we have a partial explanation of the contradiction between your diligence outside and your so-called loafing at home.

Mr. Rabin: There is some truth in what you say. But I still think the main reason is the objective circumstances. This is the problem here at the kibbutz. There is a shortage of manpower, so anyone who feels himself a partner, who does not feel that he is dealing with a factory owner who is trying to exploit him but that the plant is his also, anyone who sees the situation like that, cannot evade extra hours when the alternative is stopping production. It is true that there are people who just hang up the keys at the regular hour and care about nothing, but most of the staff work as they should.

Mrs. Rabin: On your technical staff, two out of the four keep their hours very well.

Mr. Rabin: Those two have quite different personal problems, and that is why they behave so. But the people I would call normal, more or less, are ready to put in effort, and they do care. I admit that this situation affects family life.

Kaffman: And would you ask him to stop his work?

Mrs. Rabin: God forbid!

Kaffman: But you complain so much of Michael's hard working conditions.

Mrs. Rabin: That is true, but it is not something I complain about endlessly. I just "let off steam" from time to time. Simply for selfish reasons, I ask him to come home at 3 so he can rest until 4, and then I have a fresh and active man.

Kaffman: So, what?

Mrs. Rabin: So, I let off steam; but I accept the fact that, if he finds it necessary to stay on, he knows what he is doing. He does not interfere in my work, and I do not interfere in his.

Kaffman: So, you say that, as long as he finds satisfaction in his work, then although you have to pay a certain price, you are ready to compromise.

Mrs. Rabin: More than this, I think the price I am paying is very pleasant; I do not feel I am making a sacrifice. But I think this is also the price we pay for his giving up his home and coming to live with me here at Kibbutz Regev.

Kaffman: Yes, you are from another kibbutz. You were born at Kibbutz Ma'agal.

Mrs. Rabin: That is right, and he gave up his kibbutz. He did not want to do so; I put on pressure. The reason for the pressure was mainly a family one. After all, in his family there are three more young brothers, and his parents are much younger. He is the eldest child and I am the youngest. My parents are much older and much less healthy. So, I put pressure on Michael on the subject of the family.

Kaffman: You mean that you very much wanted to stay at Kibbutz

Regev and that your special family situation helped you get your wish. But there was a difference of opinion between you, apparently quite serious. It was not easy for you to leave your home; each of you had a home at a different place, and you had to decide where to go, to your kibbutz or to his. How did you reach your decision?

Mr. Rabin: The truth is that we had a very long struggle.

Mrs. Rabin: I tried Michael's kibbutz first. We stayed at Ma'agal for a trial period of eight months, so that, later, I could better establish my feeling that we should live at my kibbutz.

Kaffman: So, you had time enough to make up your minds. How did you arrive at your common decision?

Mr. Rabin: Well, I did not want to come here, to Kibbutz Regev; but after everything is said, there are still objective circumstances. When you join a family, you must consider the parents' situation and the family in general. These are things you cannot ignore. So, you struggle, but in fact I realized that I had no choice.

Kaffman: And you had no convincing objective reason to stay at your own kibbutz?

Mr. Rabin: The only reason was that it was my home. In work and in society, I had no problems and could get along all right in either kibbutz. So it seems the family reasons were the decisive ones.

Kaffman: So, you came to Esther's kibbutz with some inner reservation and the need to overcome your objection.

Mr. Rabin: It is quite simple. I did it for Esther's sake. When you choose someone for life, you must show consideration.

Kaffman: So, you felt it was important for the proper relations between you?

Mr. Rabin: There could have been good relations at Ma'agal too, but I had the impression that the family reasons were very weighty and very important to Esther; so, finally, I agreed. To tell the truth, there were enough problems at first.

Kaffman: At the beginning of your married life?

Mr. Rabin: I do not know if it affected both of us as a couple, but it affected me personally. I did not know the Regev society too well. I knew the people, but I did not feel close to them. I had a certain feeling of strangeness, even at work. At Ma'agal my old friends used to visit us at least once a week, and here, I missed their company.

Mrs. Rabin: Yes, I knew about it, you used to tell me. But I do not think it affected our common life. I do not think it caused any family crisis, do you?

Mr. Rabin: No, the crisis was the moving from one kibbutz to another, leaving my own friends. I think my circle at Ma'agal—well, first, they were a little older than the Regev younger generation, and then, I also think they were more serious; that is my opinion, and I missed them.

Mrs. Rabin: That was also a problem which could not be avoided. It was brought about by the circumstances of changing the place where you live and the company you keep. It was not a dispute that grew out of character differences between us. I was at Ma'agal for eight months and I could not settle down to work. Not because I am a person who does not work or is not ready to accept responsibility, but because I just could not find a common language with the people there, the people who worked with me. I think this comes from the differences between our two kibbutzim, mine and Michael's.

Kaffman: Well, about your own personal relationship, you seem to have reached a fixed and agreed upon pattern of relations between you.

Mrs. Rabin: Fixed, yes, but not always agreed upon. But one learns to smooth things over, to pass them up, not to make from little things big problems. I do not think there are serious quarrels between us. After all, what could cause a serious dispute between two young people in their family life? The problem of child education?

Kaffman: Could be.

Mr. Rabin: Then we have not come to it yet; we have only one little boy.

Mrs. Rabin: It is true that I passed through a period of crisis when the boy was born. I did not like the fact that he was living at the children's house. I did not like the fact that, at night, he was away from me, under the care of the general night *metapelet* [a trained child care worker]. I was not even satisfied with the metapelet he had. But I know I live at a kibbutz and that is how life is here. I have no choice. Apart from this, in fact, I have no real complaint. At the children's house, they do the maximum for the children. Between us, it is nonsense to make an issue of the child not staying the night with me. If he slept with us at home, then we too would sleep, while at the children's house, there is always someone awake at night, near him. The metapelet hears every sound, every sneeze. So in fact, the boy is not alone, but I still feel that he is alone at night.

Kaffman: Again, the struggle between feeling and reason.

Mrs. Rabin: That is right. So I assume that it will pass with a new baby, perhaps I will get used to it. Certainly when the boy will go to kindergarten and to school, there will be other problems. But because I live at the kibbutz from choice, and not from necessity, I accept these things.

Kaffman: So the boy did not bring out any new contrasts between you. And yet, the addition of a child must have affected your family life?

Mr. Rabin: After the child was born, there was an additional thing that joined, united the family; and if he is such a lovely child, like ours, whose progress is excellent, then, of course, it adds a lot to each of us.

Mrs. Rabin: We have no problems with the boy at all. There used to be some problems. As long as the children live at the babies' house, the metapelet has no part in putting the child to bed; each mother comes to her own child. When they have moved from the babies' house, the metapelet puts them to bed for the night. Here, we suffered. Our boy was really well developed, and he was the first of all the babies to react to the fact that I went away for the day, and the first to cry when his mother went away at night. For six whole months we sat by his bed for up to an hour every evening until he dropped off to sleep. All the other children were much quieter. Some people blamed us and said that the day he started making trouble in the evening we should not have given in to him, but that we should have let him cry and left him. But I was not ready to let my child cry every evening for an hour before sleep. Perhaps if I had controlled myself and let him cry for two or three weeks, he would have overcome it too. But we sat by his side so that he could go to sleep relaxed and quiet, while I lost my own calm. I was responsible for the job assignment, at the kibbutz, and I had no patience for it. So, every evening, Michael sat with the boy. Then, when he did his reserve duty in the army, my sister came to help me, because I felt that sitting with the boy while I was a bundle of nerves could not relax him. I was very tense because of my job, being in a hurry to finish my affairs, and I would have only harmed him. So, until Michael returned from the army, I took care of the boy only partly, assisted partly by my father and my sister. But when Michael was at home, this was his job; with me, it took the boy an hour to get to sleep, and with Michael, only twenty minutes. With me, he used to play and be unruly; he took advantage of me.

Mr. Rabin: From the day he moved to the toddlers' house and putting him to bed became the metapelet's responsibility, all the problems were over. He goes to the metapelet; says "good-bye, Mommy; good-bye, Daddy." He does not need anything and anybody.

Mrs. Rabin: The change was so drastic and surprising from the first day we brought him in the evening back to his new house; he sat down at the table with the metapelet, looked at a picture book, and that was it. No "Mommy," no "Daddy," nothing. I had a natural urge to disappear the moment he turned his head, but of course, I do not do it. I call him, say, "Good-bye, Mother is going." The boy knows I am going; he sees me going; and there are no problems.

Kaffman: Certainly, I think this is the best way, to accustom the child, not by suddenly disappearing, because then his confidence is shaken, but the way you did it, "immunizing" the boy against parting, gradually and naturally. I think, if I got it right, your common care of the boy brought an additional subject about which to talk; it did not add differences or disputes, but on the contrary—

Mrs. Rabin: No, there are no differences about the boy. Even when he was born, it was planned and agreed between us. I wanted to go out and study; I expected an answer from the university; and when it turned out that I was not going, it was clear that we had nothing to wait for with a baby. Now I am going to the university at Jerusalem for a whole year, and I am leaving Michael alone to be both father and mother for six days a week.

Kaffman: With complete confidence.

Mrs. Rabin: Yes, sure. It hurts a little, but—

Mr. Rabin: It will be difficult. I see now how the boy reacts when I go to the army; so it is sure to be much harder when his mother will leave for a whole year. But I think we will get over it.

Mrs. Rabin: The main problem is that Jerusalem is so far away, and my schedule includes studies on Friday too and late every evening of the week. At the kibbutz, it has never happened before that the mother of a small child should leave on Sunday morning and return on Friday afternoon.

Kaffman: I wonder how you reached such a decision, I mean, for Esther to go out and study for a year.

Mr. Rabin: I do not know whether you can regard this as a problem. It was quite obvious to both of us that Esther must study. The only question was whether I could take care of the boy and be completely free for the hours with him. If this were possible, then, there would be no problem. Postponing the studies until the boy grew up would mean having to wait for many years, because later there probably will be some more children. So, it is better for her to leave when she has one child, rather than two. I could see no better alternative.

Mrs. Rabin: Perhaps I could have postponed my studies for two more years, until the boy will be four or five. Perhaps we made a mistake about it, but we are not sorry.

Kaffman: It seems to me quite legitimate to wish and strive for self-fulfillment, especially when you rely on Michael to do the parents' job, in spite of the difficulties.

Mrs. Rabin: Quite. It was difficult for me too when he was in the army. It was difficult to face the boy's reaction. But you must decide what is preferable. After all, the boy is not left alone; he stays with his father.

Kaffman: I see that decisions about your common affairs are made according to clear and reasonable considerations, according to the rule that in the end you always reach an agreement, and in controversial matters reason finally overcomes emotion.

Mrs. Rabin: Every time I start such a controversy, I always think that, in fact, I am to blame, because I exaggerate my complaints. When I consider things impartially, then I am convinced there is no proportion between my accusations and the actual facts.

Kaffman: If I got it right, you said that your need to quarrel and complain is not so related to what he does or fails to do.

Mrs. Rabin: That is right. Quite often my outburst against Michael stems from an unconnected matter altogether—outside influence, my reaction to all sorts of things.

Mr. Rabin: Sometimes you get angry with somebody, about things at work, and then you have an outburst at home. In these cases, you are not really angry with me, but your anger finds an outlet with me.

Mrs. Rabin: Because I have nobody else?

Mr. Rabin: So, you unburden yourself of your anger and it passes. We could say I am a help with it. But there are cases—mm, well, cases when I receive a direct frontal attack. There are from time to time little eruptions like that, but we have learned not to bear a grudge and it comes and goes on, and that is it.

Mrs. Rabin: In the first years, there were many problems around this subject. I would say, "You keep so much to yourself that I do not know what you are holding inside you." Today, it is no problem. Now I do not need him to tell me what he feels inside.

Mr. Rabin: Yes, I also feel that each of us knows the other better, and she is more willing to meet me halfway. Esther—

Mrs. Rabin: This I want to hear again.

Mr. Rabin: Esther helps me in concrete things too. Every time I feel better cooperation between us. For example, I had a job at the kibbutz and one day I was away, so Esther did for me various tasks. She helps me many times.

Mrs. Rabin: I enjoy being your secretary, but not only a secretary. I like learning the work.

Mr. Rabin: She is also a housewife with many unhousewifelike qualities. For example, she can put nails in the wall, use a drill, and things like that.

Mrs. Rabin: It is not nice to say it myself, but I can manage alone when it is necessary.

Kaffman: Fine. Now I get the impression that throughout the years you have improved the means of communication between you.

Mrs. Rabin: That is what I think. For example, this matter of Michael's silences has not been an issue for some years now.

Mr. Rabin: We have no problem of communication on any subject at all.

Mrs. Rabin: I think we can talk about every subject without difficulty.

Mr. Rabin: I think so too.

Mrs. Rabin: There was a period when it was not like that, but for some years now there are no problems.

Kaffman: Do you have an understanding in sexual matters too?

Mrs. Rabin: Yes, certainly, this is one of the most important subjects. The problems here existed long ago, when we were very young; but they were caused, not by the relations between us, but by the relations between us and the "public."

Mr. Rabin: We were under the constant watch and control of our group and of people—teachers and relatives—who put pressure on us to wait.

Mrs. Rabin: So this background created many tensions, which affected us both—between us—but all this has become quite unimportant today. It had no effect on the development of harmonious relations and mutual adjustment in sexual matters.

Kaffman: You say your respective families, one at Ma'agal and the other at Regev, tried to influence you. Perhaps we had better hear a little about your families now. You have said a great deal about the influence of the group, of society, of public opinion, and so far, this subject of your families has not come up. Does the family at the kibbutz have any meaning?

Mrs. Rabin: Yes, quite considerable. But I would like Michael to start with his own family. It would be easier for me this way.

Mr. Rabin: As it happens, my parents did not contribute too much to the relations between myself and Esther. Perhaps it was just because I felt their objections that I was drawn closer to her. My parents always tried to hide their objection, but it was very obvious. Between me and my parents there were no open talks on friendship, love. I never heard my parents talk between themselves about emotional matters. In this respect, relations between me and my parents were very distant. On the other hand, they tried very hard to give me and my brothers everything material, so we should have special food and the utmost comfort in our room. But there were no free talks and close relations between us.

Kaffman: What could have been the cause?

Mr. Rabin: I think it was the same in their homes. And, sometimes, they used to tell us about the time right after the kibbutz was founded—I was a boy then—when it was taken for granted that any problems of the child or the adolescent should be taken care of only inside the educational framework. But all this was years ago; in the meantime, the attitude has changed, and now nobody tries to take away the parents' right to talk with their children about their problems or to show an interest in them. But I see that nothing changed in the relations between my parents and my younger brothers. It has nothing to do with the system. They apparently find it difficult to get closer. Today, I treat these matters differently. I am much more free with them; but at the time, relations were different in this respect, because I too took no initiative to try to get closer to them. A large part of my problems was unknown to them. Apart from conversation, we had everything: games, toys, sometimes we used to go to town to the movies and to see places.

Kaffman: Apparently, this was the only way they knew of expressing their love.

Mr. Rabin: Even now, they still send us regularly cakes and special dishes, but there is still no possibility of talking about personal problems. On the other hand, communication with my brothers is good.

Kaffman: Perhaps this was one of the reasons you were attracted to Esther. With her and with her parents you saw exactly what you felt you were missing in your parents' room.

Mrs. Rabin: No, the first initiative between us was mine.

Kaffman: Really?

Mrs. Rabin: Yes, certainly. But it was a small detail, I think. I think that the root of the problems between parents and children is the differences in intellectual level. I think that this is a main cause of family problems. The intellectual level is not enough. Your father is on a little higher level, but your mother is just "a Jewish mother" and nothing more. It is hard to understand, but if I compare my mother to yours—my mother finished university in Poland, continued studying at the university here in Israel, and all her life she has been dealing with education and teaching. In the nature of things, she is much more educated, involved in things; she meets people. My parents are more people of the world. They are much more receptive; they read much more, get around. Your parents live their lives within their four walls. Your father is more open in this respect, but you have a good-hearted mother. She is so kind that, sometimes, it is hard to bear. She surrounds you with material wealth and warmth of heart, but these are not enough.

Kaffman: You attach much more importance than does Michael to the matter of cultural background, cultural interests, while he reacts to two things: he is very sorry about the cultural poverty within his parents' room, but in addition, he feels there is some difficulty in communication.

Mrs. Rabin: The two things overlap. I know many families where the cultural level is not high but emotional contact is very deep and strong. That is true. But I consider this point about differences in level as more important than the question of collective education at the kibbutz, where parents and children live in separate houses. My mother too brought up her children like that. She had my elder sister eight years before Michael was even born. He is the eldest son in his family. I have a sister who is thirty-four, and my mother brought her up under much more strict conditions in all things that had to do with handing over the job of looking after the children and educating them from the parents to the child care workers. But in spite of this, we grew up different, and the communication between me and my sister and between my parents is quite different, compared to Michael's family. With us, family meetings are much more intellectual; they are simply much more interesting, but there is no human contact expressed in heart-to-heart talk. I feel no urge to talk with my parents about intimate matters. It is probably the result of a certain education. I do not know who is to blame for it, but it is a fact. Perhaps the explanation is that I have an elder sister who replaced my mother in many respects. I have excellent communication with my sister.

Kaffman: Including the possibility of discussing the intimate matters which you keep from your parents?

Mrs. Rabin: Not everything, only in part. I do not feel any need to always let someone into my problems. But my sister and I are very close. Relations between us are very open and free.

Kaffman: It sounds as though your relationship with your respective families is mainly the relations between you and your siblings.

Mr. Rabin: But at the same time, we also keep regular and proper relations with both of our families.

Mrs. Rabin: Relations are good, but no one interferes in the other's affairs. Actually, I think that I interfere in my parents' affairs more than they do in mine. More than once I have interfered in their arguments. Well, of course, they argue in front of me so that is understandable. My sister and I many times mix up in our parents' arguments, even take sides. I think this is quite natural.

Kaffman: And this is more or less regularly? I see there is some sort of a fixed pattern in your mutual behavior. Now what about the wider family, are there any fixed patterns?

Mrs. Rabin: With your family, Michael, I do not think there are any regular responses, but with us, there are. The situation is unpleasant, because my sister and I side with our father much more than with our mother. Even when she is often right, we do not support her. It has become a sort of united front against her, rightly or wrongly. I think that our father just understands us better, but these things are much more emotional than they are rational. That is how relations developed during the years. Sometimes, I am very much aware that Mother is right and I still continue supporting the opposite side.

Kaffman: You probably have your own explanation of this special situation.

Mrs. Rabin: Father has always been the strong member of the family. He always played the chief role. I do not remember much about the relations between myself and my parents when I was very young. Mostly, I have memories of recent years. Usually, with my own affairs, I turn to Father and not to Mother. For example, I find it easier to leave my son with him, not that I trust my mother less, heaven forbid, but it seems Father gets along better with the boy than does Mother. Well, this again could be just prejudice.

Kaffman: If I understand it correctly, the way your family works, I mean you in relation to Michael, is quite different from, perhaps even the exact opposite from, the way your mother acted in relation to your father.

Mrs. Rabin: That is correct.

Mr. Rabin: I think that her father is younger in spirit, so he is easier to approach. Esther's character, I think, is like her father's, and the sense of humor is similar too. Esther's impulsiveness also comes from her father. The mother is different.

Mrs. Rabin: And of the entire family, the person who treats Mother in the nicest way is Michael. He is patient with her, always ready to listen.

Mr. Rabin: These two daughters react a little too much to their mother. Esther has already said that it is not a question of right or wrong. They do not consider each thing on its own merit; instead, there is a fixed attitude that Mother is like this and Father is like that. I do not like it, because I am accustomed to a different attitude at home. We treat our parents a little differently.

Kaffman: Both of you have mentioned the special closeness and feelings of identification between Esther and her father, which has brought about this united front. On his side, Michael is a moderating influence in the relationship between Esther and her mother. He helps your mother. Now, Michael claims that the situation is different in his family. What happens there?

Mrs. Rabin: I think that Michael partly inherited his mother's virtues. Not her reserve against the world, but he inherited her quiet, her calm. She is always good and smiling.

Kaffman: That is interesting. Each of you has brought into your common family one of his parents, or rather, the traits of one of his parents. Esther has brought in her father and you have brought in your mother.

Mr. Rabin: Yes, there is something in what you say.

Kaffman: Somehow, things repeat themselves, in a new and corrected edition. We are getting close to the end of our interview. Well, to sum up your years of attachment, it can be said that—

Mrs. Rabin: For my part, I think that it could not have been better than it has been during these years, because I have everything; in fact, I do not need any more than that. It is true that I sometimes have a feeling of jealousy when I visit my sister at Kibbutz Ganim. I see one of her neighbors there, and he is an ideal husband, a perfect husband. What do I mean? The wife has a whip in her hand. For example, she

says, "It is Thursday today and we are going to thoroughly clean the
house." She does not care whether he is tired or not. He accepts
this without argument and, apparently, without resentment. Then he
starts taking off the screens from the windows, scrubbing the house.
They look happy, seem to have a good life. But I am contented
with what I have. I do not think I would have felt happy if I had such
an obedient husband. Still, it does not stop my jealous feeling when
I see this woman and everything that her husband has done for her,
while I never know when Michael will do for me what I have asked him
to do.

Kaffman: So, you would not like to exchange Michael for that
perfect husband? But perhaps you only say so for me to hear.

Mrs. Rabin: Michael knows it very well. Look, it has been quite a
few years now. I had more than one chance to change him, and I did
not want to.

Kaffman: You are silent, Michael, What is your summation?

Mr. Rabin: Perhaps Esther is considered at the kibbutz as a little of
a difficult wife, but with it all, I do not know whether there are here
many better families as far as open personal relations are concerned. I
do not think I have seen many girls with whom you could achieve
such a relationship. Perhaps I am wrong, but that is how it seems to
me. I am not talking about simple erotic and passing intimate relations,
but about a permanent bond of friendship, the possibility of talking
with each other, the mutually fair attitude, the quality of conversation
and the emotional affinity. When I think of all the girls at the kibbutz
that I know, then I feel that Esther is one of the most loyal, considered as a wife who follows you not only at times of quarrel but
throughout the years.

Mrs. Rabin: And we still have quite a long way to go.

Kaffman: And perhaps one last question: if you were asked to "sell"
the secret of a more or less harmonious married life, even with some
frictions here and some differences there, if you wanted to pass on
a little of your experience to others, what would you say?

Mrs. Rabin: I am very weak on recipes; that is what Michael's mother
is good at. It is hard for me to say. I would certainly not be the one to
give anybody advice on how to live his life. It is a difficult problem,
but I will tell you, I think the secret of our balanced life is Michael's
character. If I had a husband with a character like mine, then I would
have a very hard life. I think Michael's character brings to our life its
balance and stability, because after all I can depend on him. I know

that as much as I act madly and unrestrainedly, he will never lose his temper because of things that drive me into a rage. I think it is something like the coexistence of two persons of complementary tempers. But that is not a recipe you can pass on to someone else.

Mr. Rabin: The relationship created between us is very personal. It is difficult to "sell" it to other couples.

Kaffman: It sounds quite simple: the complementing of characters between a man and a woman. Is not that enough? Then perhaps we could use computers to match the couples, and then married life would be stable and harmonious.

Mrs. Rabin: No, I do not think it is as simple as that. The right choice of partners is not enough. Later, there is a lot to learn throughout the married life itself. I will tell you, during our years together we have learned to know each other. It sounds simple, but it is not easy to know and respect each other. In fact, that is the secret of success in our married life, there is no other secret. It has taken years to discover it.

Mr. Rabin: And it will take more years.

Mrs. Rabin: Could be. There are still many problems which we have not yet come across. Time will probably bring new tests. We will live and see them. I hope we stand them well.

Mr. Rabin: So do I.

Kaffman: And I too. I want to thank you again for wrestling for almost three hours with the problems brought up in this interview. You have really done your best, with honesty, and I think that this conversation can help anyone interested in learning how relations are built between partners living together for years.

The reader can draw the parallels on his own between the Wagners and the Rabins. Although the families live in different cultures, they have faced similar problems in forming a family—drawing boundaries around the new structure, dealing with in-laws, relating to friends, and rearing children. The tasks take different forms in the two societies, but the diversity of cultures only highlights the essential similarity of the process.

5 Therapeutic Implications of a Structural Approach

In essence, the structural approach to families is based on the concept that a family is more than the individual biopsychodynamics of its members. Family members relate according to certain arrangements, which govern their transactions. These arrangements, though usually not explicitly stated or even recognized, form a whole—the structure of the family. The reality of the structure is of a different order from the reality of the individual members.

Family structure is not an entity immediately available to the observer. The therapist's data and his diagnoses are achieved experientially in the process of joining the family. He hears what the family members tell him about the way that they experience reality. But he also observes the way that family members relate to him and to each other. The therapist analyzes the transactional field in which he and the family are meeting, in order to make a structural diagnosis.

The therapist asks himself a number of questions. For example, who is the family spokesman? If the father is acting as spokesman, what does this mean? Who selected him to make the presentation—to bear the main responsibility for the first contact with a significant extrafamilial person? Is he taking the spokesman's position because he is the executive head of the family? Or is the mother the true executive leader, who is ceding her power temporarily to the father because of some implicit rule about the proper role of men? What is she doing while her husband talks? Is she tacitly seconding his communications, or is she interfering with them by verbal or nonverbal means?

Further, is the content of the verbal communications supported or contradicted by the family's behavior? Is what takes place in the session typical of other moments in the family's life? Would the affective tone of family interaction change if the composition of the session were different? Are the transactions currently underway in the session more significant than those that occurred earlier in the session?

While the therapist is responding to events as they occur in the session, he is also making observations and posing questions. He starts to pinpoint transactional patterns and boundaries, and to make hypotheses about which patterns are functional and which are dysfunctional. He is beginning to derive a family map.

A family map is an organizational scheme. It does not represent the richness of family transactions any more than a map represents the richness of a territory. It is static, whereas the family is constantly in motion. But the family map is a powerful simplification device, which allows the therapist to organize the diverse material that he is getting. The map allows him to formulate hypotheses about areas within the family that function well and about other areas that may be dysfunctional. It also helps him to determine the therapeutic goals.

The function of such maps was described by Claude Lévi-Strauss in another context: "One of the peculiarities of the small societies which we study is that each constitutes, as it were, a ready-made experiment . . . On the other hand, these societies are alive, and we have neither the time nor the means to manipulate them . . . we find our experiments already prepared but they are uncontrollable . . . therefore . . . we attempt to replace them with models, systems of symbols which preserve the characteristic properties of the experiment, but which we can manipulate."[1] Like the anthropologist, the structural family therapist uses a map to organize the material he is gathering.

PROBING WITHIN THE THERAPEUTIC SYSTEM

While the therapist is gathering material for a structural map, he is also introducing experimental probes. In a sense, his very presence is a probe, because the family is organizing in relation to him. But in addition, he can impose tasks designed to probe significant aspects of family structure.

The family therapist regards himself as an acting and reacting member of the therapeutic system. In order to join the family, he emphasizes the aspects of his personality and experience that are syntonic with the family's. But he also retains the freedom to be spontaneous in his experimental probes.

This use of self is very different from that of the psychodynamically oriented therapist. The premises of psychodynamic therapy are that change occurs in the individual through cognitive-affective re-encounter with the introjected past. This re-encounter occurs through a symbolic relationship with the therapist. Consequently, the individual therapist is taught to keep his personal responses in check. He must have a capacity for controlling his impulses and for watchful observation of his internal processes. He must discriminate between his objective responses and the responses issuing from his own past that are evoked by the current behavior of the patient through countertransference. He develops a capacity for passive observation and learns to appraise his spontaneous responses with caution. His role is to force the patient to look at himself and his relationship to the significant figures of his past. His emphasis is on the exploration of the conflictual past and on interpreting it in the present.

The premises of change are different in family therapy. Change is seen as occurring through the process of the therapist's affiliation with the family and his restructuring of the family in a carefully planned way, so as to transform dysfunctional transactional patterns. If he has been able to affiliate with a family and feels the pressures of the family system, he does not need to guard against spontaneous responses, for those responses will probably be syntonic with that system. If they are not, they can be valuable as experimental probes.

The only family structure immediately available to a therapist is the dysfunctional structure. One of the tasks he faces is to probe that structure and to locate areas of possible flexibility and change. His input highlights parts of the family structure that have been submerged. Structural alternatives that have lain quiescent become active. If the therapist then has the flexibility to disengage himself and observe the effect of his probes, they will clarify his diagnostic picture of the family.

A family usually dismisses probes that are not syntonic with the family system. When they do respond, however, one of three things may happen. The family may assimilate the therapist's input to its previous transactional patterns without difficulty. This produces learning but not growth. The family may also respond by accommodating itself, either by expanding its transactional patterns or by activating alternative patterns. Finally, the family may respond to the therapist's input as if to a completely novel situation. In this case the probe has become a restructuring intervention. If the family does not reject it, there will be an increase of stress in the system. The homeostasis of the family will be unbalanced, opening the way for transformation.

Two examples will clarify how the therapist probes and evaluates his probes within a therapeutic system. A family composed of a mother, father, and four children is beginning therapy. The presenting problem, or identified patient, is a ten-year-old boy who steals and plays hookey.

The mother signals to the father to start the session. While he is talking, she silently monitors the behavior of the five-year-old daughter (D) and the seven-year-old son (S). She interrupts her husband to qualify a statement. Then she signals the fourteen-year-old daughter to express her point of view and interrupts her to tell her to talk honestly to the therapist. While the daughter is talking, she watches her mother, and at one point she asks her mother the date of the incident she is describing.

From his observations so far, the therapist (Th) can tentatively map this family's structure. In his first diagnostic hypothesis, the mother appears as the central switchboard, through whom family operations must be routed (Fig. 11).

Fig. 11

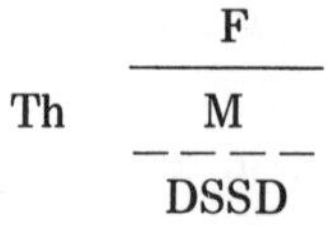

$$\text{Th} \quad \frac{\overline{\text{F}}}{\underset{\text{DSSD}}{\text{M}}}$$

Now the therapist probes to test the flexibility of the family's internal boundaries. He asks the mother to move away from the children and keep silent. This task enables him to observe how competent the father is with his children, and what capacity for autonomy the children have when their mother becomes less active. If the father can interact comfortably with the children, the therapist will hypothesize a clear parental subsystem boundary and probe elsewhere in his search for dysfunctional areas within the family. However, if the father is ineffective and the children cannot deal with him autonomously, the therapist will hypothesize an inappropriately rigid boundary that separates father from children and keeps the mother overinvolved with the children. This hypothesis delimits a dysfunctional area, implies a therapeutic goal, and suggests certain steps that may help to reach that goal.

In another family, the identified patient (IP) is a fifteen-year-old diabetic girl who refuses to follow a proper diet, falsifies her urine tests, and cannot be trusted to administer her own insulin shots. The mother, the father, the identified patient, and her younger sister are seen in family therapy.

The father starts the session. He describes the onset of his daughter's illness and how it affected the family. When he finishes, he touches his wife and says, "Now you talk." The therapist says jokingly that it looks like a relay race. The family laughs. The mother describes how her daughter's illness affects her. Among other things, she says she must always watch to make sure the daughter eats the right things. As the mother talks, she maintains eye contact with all the other family members. The diabetic girl interrupts her mother to describe her eating problems. But while she is talking, she interrupts herself with long pauses, which are filled by the mother.

The therapist intervenes to ask the younger daughter how she activates her mother. He points out that the father activated her by touching her and giving her a task, and the older daughter activated her by creating long pauses for the mother to fill. The younger daughter replies that she does not think she activates her mother. At this point the therapist has the basic ingredients for a map, in which the mother is central and overinvolved with the identified patient (Fig. 12).

Fig. 12

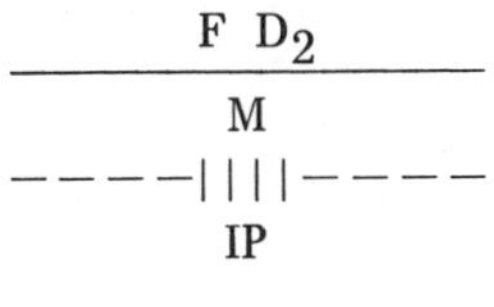

$$\begin{array}{c} \underline{\hspace{1cm} F \quad D_2 \hspace{1cm}} \\ M \\ ----|\,|\,|\,|---- \\ IP \end{array}$$

Now the therapist probes further. He imposes a rule. No one is to talk for anyone else, and no one may guess another family member's thoughts or feelings. Then the therapist asks the father if there is any other problem in the family. The father says that his wife feels anxious when he is away from home. The therapist points out that the father has broken the rule, just as the father begins to say, "Oh, I'm not supposed to talk for anyone else." This is a good prognostic sign, indicating that the father has enough resources to make use of the therapist's input.

The older daughter says that her father does not take enough interest in her. She complains that he did not attend her school concert. The younger daughter says he will not help her with her homework. At this point a new map may be drawn, in which the mother is in coalition with the daughters against the father, who is peripheral (Fig. 13).

Fig. 13
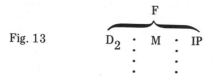

$$D_2 \cdot M \cdot IP$$

These two maps imply a goal: to define a boundary around the spouse subsystem that will increase the distance between the mother and the identified patient and will draw the peripheral father closer into the family. Accordingly, the therapist rebukes both girls for breaking the rule. He tells them that they took over their mother's complaint about their father's not spending enough time at home, turning a wife's complaint about her husband into a daughters' complaint about their father.

Later, the husband and wife begin to argue about finances as well as difficulties the husband is having with his job. When the wife criticizes him, the older daughter intervenes, saying that she has some savings the family could use. The mother begins arguing with the daughter, abandoning her argument with her husband. Now that spouse conflict has arisen, the map takes on a new cast (Fig. 14).

Fig. 14
$$\frac{F-||-M}{D_1 \, D_2} \quad \text{becomes} \quad \frac{F \vdots M - || - D_1}{D_2}$$

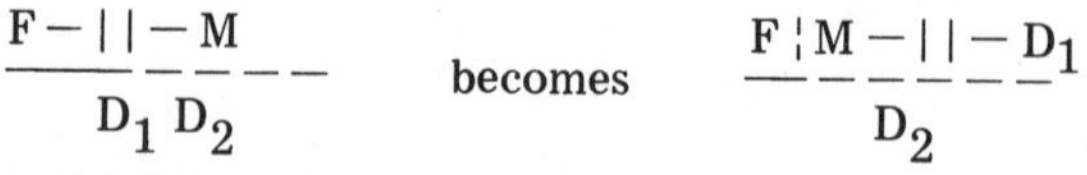

In this family, the spouses detour conflict by transforming a spouse conflict into a conflict between the mother or father and the daughter. Again the map suggests a goal and a pathway to that goal. The therapist asks both daughters to move their chairs close to his and sit with their backs to their parents. He asks the parents to resume their argument and continue it to a conclusion. They do so, and both girls seem to enjoy the artificial seating arrangement.

The first session suggests an initial mapping of the family that gives the therapist a goal for the family and indicates some steps to achieve that goal. Further sessions and subsequent assessments will qualify the map, refine it, and make it more accurate.

Frequently encountered family models—such as the extended family, the family with a parental child, and the family in a transitional situation—provide further illustrations of the application of structural analysis. No family model is inherently normal or abnormal, functional or dysfunctional. A family's differentiation is idiosyncratic, related to its own composition, developmental stage, and subculture, and any model is workable. But every model has inherent weaknesses, and these may be the parts that give way when the family's coping capacity becomes exhausted.

THE EXTENDED FAMILY

The extended family model is a form well adapted to situations of stress and scarcity. It is therefore a highly significant model in many poverty-stricken families. Functions can be shared. One member can care for the children while all the other adults work to support the total family. Household chores and other tasks can be shared. A woman can take her sister's children to the clinic for a checkup when she takes her own. The companionship and multiple sources of help and support available within the extended family frequently make it the only possible form for a family in conditions of scarcity.

The extended family, in particular the "urban matriarchal" extended family, received a great deal of publicity from propaganda generated by the helping professions during the "war on poverty." As a result, a therapist may be preconditioned to pounce on this form as inherently pathogenic. Careful structural mapping, however, may show that the system is functioning adequately.

In other cases, an extended family may run into problems because of the difficulty of allocating responsibility clearly. Because of the complexity of the family unit, there may be a number of vague boundaries, which creates confusion and stress.

For instance, a family comes into therapy because of the youngest daughter, aged ten, who does not obey, wanders away from home, and comes home from school very late without having let her family know where she was. The mother called the therapist, so the first contact with the family is with the mother and five children. In the first session, the therapist observes that the mother has problems of control with all five children (Fig. 15).

Fig. 15   Th   M
                                   · · · · · · ·
                                   SSSDD

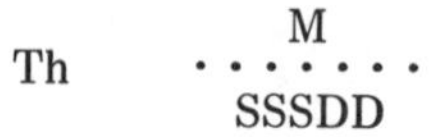

The therapist then spreads the problem beyond the identified patient by pointing out the mother's difficulty with all of her children. He thereby forms a therapeutic contract, which establishes the agreement that therapy will include working with the identified patient, helping the mother to control all of her children better, and finding supports for her. When he finds out that a grandmother also lives with the family, he urges her to come to the next session.

When the grandmother is present, it is obvious that she is the executive head of the family. The mother's power and competence disappear in the presence of her own mother (Fig. 16). The therapist's

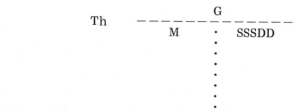

Fig. 16

map of this parenting structure orients his restructuring interventions toward the goal of joining the mother and grandmother together in the parental subsystem in a position of complementarity and mutual support (Fig. 17).

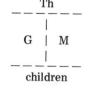

Fig. 17
The Therapeutic
Goal

Many strategies can be used to achieve this goal. The grandmother can go behind a one-way mirror to watch her daughter parenting the children (Fig. 18). The one-way mirror forms a boundary which allows

Fig. 18   G
                    ─────────────────   (one-way mirror)
                             Th M
                    ─ ─ ─ ─ ─ ─ ─ ─ ─
                         children

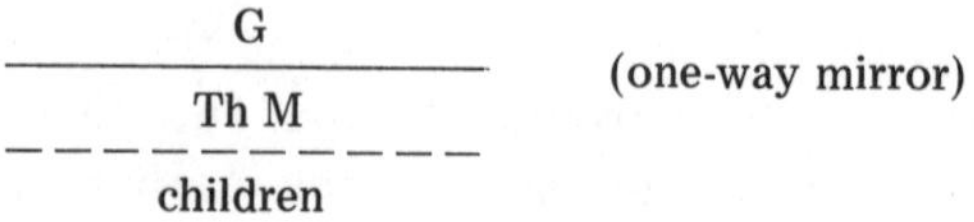

the feeling of participation without input. The therapist can keep the grandmother in the room, using himself to block her taking over (Fig. 19). He can hold sessions with only the grandmother and

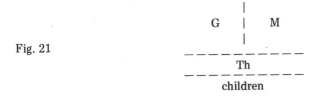

Fig. 19

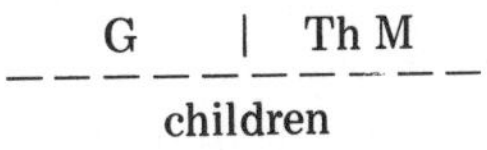

Fig. 20

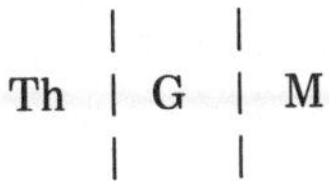

mother, including himself in an alliance of executives (Fig. 20). Or he can position himself between the adults and the children, clarifying the boundary around the mother and grandmother, and at the same time serving as a model of executive parenting behavior for both subsystems, parental and child (Fig. 21).

```
                        |
            G   |   M
                |
Fig. 21     _ _ _ _ _ _ _ _ _
                Th
            _ _ _ _ _ _ _ _ _
              children
```

These strategies are only a few examples of the many possible approaches to achieving this therapeutic goal in this type of family structure. The therapist may use all of these strategies as well as others at different times in therapy. But whatever approach he initially chooses in his attempt to restructure the family will have an impact on the family's responses to him. It will open certain pathways of intervention, and close others.

THE FAMILY WITH A PARENTAL CHILD

The allocation of parental power to a child is a natural arrangement in large families, in single-parent families, or in families where both parents work. The system can function well. The younger children are cared for, and the parental child can develop responsibility, competence, and autonomy beyond his years.

A family with a parental child structure may run into difficulty, however, if the delegation of authority is not explicit or if the parents abdicate, leaving the child to become the main source of guidance, control, and decisions. In such a case, the demands on the parental child can clash with his own childhood needs and exceed his ability to cope with them.

The Gordens (Chapter 11) illustrate the problem. In this family the boundary between mother and ten-year-old parental child has become diffuse. They form a tight subsystem with a boundary impermeable to the other children. Authority has been clearly delegated, but the demands on the parental child have outstripped his ability to perform (Fig. 22). The identified patient—the older daughter, aged seven—is a

Fig. 22

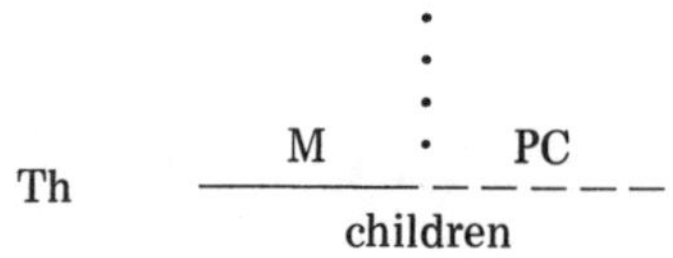

firesetter. Because of the inappropriately rigid boundary, reinforced by the activity of the parental child, the mother scapegoats the identified patient instead of supporting her (Fig. 23).

Fig. 23

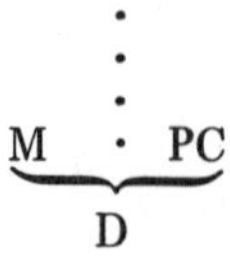

In this case, the therapeutic goal is to realign the family in such a way that the parental child can still help the mother. The boundary between mother and parental child has to be clarified. The boundary between mother and other children has to be modified to allow them direct access to her. The parental child has to be returned to the sibling subgroup, though he maintains his position of leadership and junior executive power (Fig. 24).

Fig. 24
The Therapeutic
Goal

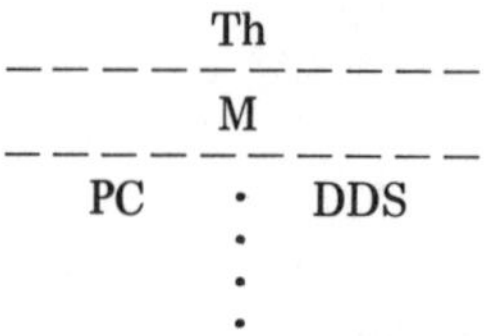

THE FAMILY IN TRANSITIONAL SITUATIONS

Temporary Loss. Although a family may be stressed in all kinds of transitional situations, this is particularly true in cases of separation and return. When one of the parents leaves the family, one set of adaptations must be negotiated. If the husband leaves the wife, some changes take place (Fig. 25). If he returns, the changes must be reversed.

Fig. 25

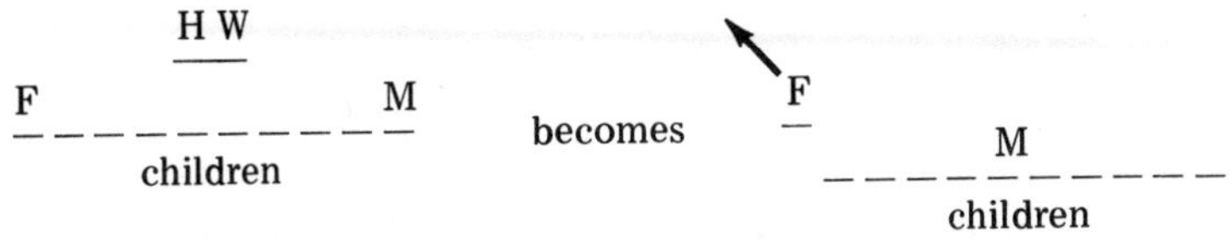

$$\underset{\text{children}}{\text{F} \text{----------} \text{M}} \quad \overset{\text{H W}}{} \quad \text{becomes} \quad \underset{}{\text{F}} \quad \underset{\text{children}}{\text{M} \text{----------}}$$

Spouse transactions are interrupted and must reform. Parental transactions change and must be renegotiated. The returning parent must form new relationships with the children. Three subsystems disappear, then reappear, and must be absorbed as part of the functioning of the newly reformed system.

Sometimes such transitional negotiations can be blocked. The affected transactional patterns then become weak links. For example, a family calls the therapist because they are having a problem with their ten-year-old daughter, who, they say, is promiscuous. When they come to the session, they spend most of the time talking about the problems of their eight-year-old son, who is disobedient.

The therapist observes a family structure that seems to include the mother and children in a coalition against the father. The children interrupt spouse transactions, and the father is excluded from parenting transactions (Fig. 26).

Fig. 26   Th   F $\left\{ \begin{array}{c} \text{H} \overset{......}{} \text{W} \\ \underset{\text{children}}{\text{M}} \end{array} \right.$

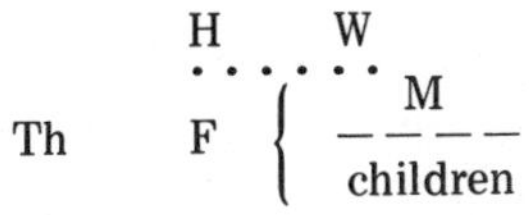

In the session, the father volunteers the information that four years ago he began three years in jail. Apparently some of the problems of readapting to the father's presence have not been solved. A chronic transitional situation has developed, in which dysfunctional structures have arisen.

In this family the therapeutic goal is to increase the strength of the boundary around husband and wife, excluding the children from spouse transactions and allowing the father to take on parental functions. In order to achieve this, the therapist may affiliate with the father, increasing his salience in the family (Fig. 27). He may block

Fig. 27   Th $\overbrace{\text{M} \vdots \text{children}}^{}$ becomes $\begin{array}{c} \text{Th} == \text{F M} \\ \overline{-----} \\ \text{children} \end{array}$

$\underbrace{}_{\text{F}}$

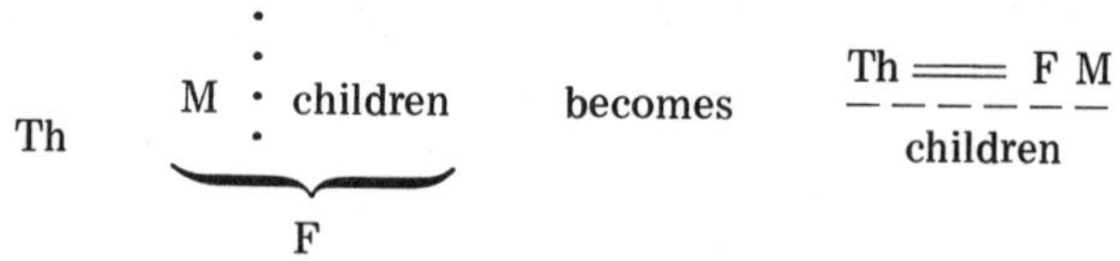

the mother-children transactions, perhaps by conducting therapy with them alone or by blocking the mother's movements in the session (Fig. 28). These tactics will open the boundary between the father and the children and move the mother toward the father.

Fig. 28   M $\Big|$ $\begin{array}{c} \text{Th} == \text{F} \\ --||-- \\ \text{children} \end{array}$

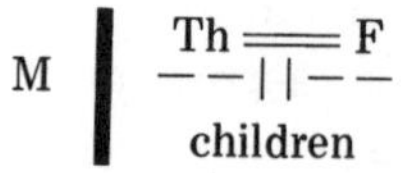

Finally, he can join the mother and father in a coalition against the children, attacking them for disobedience, or he can use the tactic of pointing up the parents' incompetence with the children. Either technique makes the parents join to form an effective parental unit (Fig. 29).

Fig. 29 $\overbrace{\text{Th F M}}^{}$
$\underbrace{}_{\text{children}}$

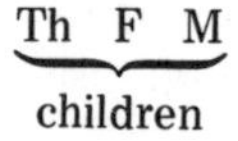

Any one of these methods may help the family to solve the problem that arose when transitional negotiations around the reinclusion of the father were blocked. Similar problems can arise when transitions around the permanent loss of a family member, as through death or divorce, are blocked.

Divorce. When a couple divorces, the man is usually better able to disengage than the woman. The social conditions which decree that the mother should take the children produce, on her part, a continuing commitment to the previous system.

For example, a family comes into therapy because the older daughter, aged sixteen, has become depressed and withdrawn. The parents were divorced six months earlier, and the father is now living alone. The mother suggests that the therapist arrange a session with her and her ex-husband, so they can discuss some of the things they might do for their children. This meeting is held, and the divorced couple fight bitterly throughout it. Meeting with the therapist immediately afterward, the mother says that she is impressed by how detached she felt. But she tells the therapist that she thinks her ex-husband is very sick, and she would like the therapist to take him into individual therapy.

The mother's contention that she feels disengaged from her ex-husband is challenged by several factors. Two of the children, who were very attached to their father, now refuse any contact with him. The younger children visit their father but express great unhappiness with the situation. And the mother wants the therapist who is working with her and her children to take her husband into treatment.

A map of the situation suggests that the negotiations around the ex-husband's leaving have been blocked by the mother's and children's commitment to the old system. In such a situation, to see the ex-husband with his wife and children would only reinforce the strong antagonism between the former spouses. Analysis of the systems indicates that the unit to treat is the mother and children without the father. The therapist can then arrange a few sessions with the father and children without the mother as a way of developing negotiations that will make it possible for the children and their father to maintain a relationship, although he is peripheral to the old system (Fig. 30).

Fig. 30
The Therapeutic
Goal

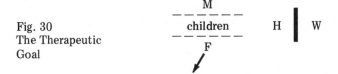

Chronic Boundary Problems. Still other families may come into therapy because of chronic boundary problems related to the negotiation of stresses in one subsystem through other subsystems. In an effectively functioning family, this type of negotiation is possible because the system is governed by clear yet flexible boundaries. However, dysfunctional sets may appear if one subsystem always uses the same nonmember to diffuse subsystem conflicts. This is seen most commonly when parents use a child to detour or deflect spouse conflicts. The boundary between the parental subsystem and the child becomes diffuse, and the boundary around the parents-child triad, which should be diffuse, becomes inappropriately rigid (Fig. 31). This type of structure is called a rigid triad.

Fig. 31

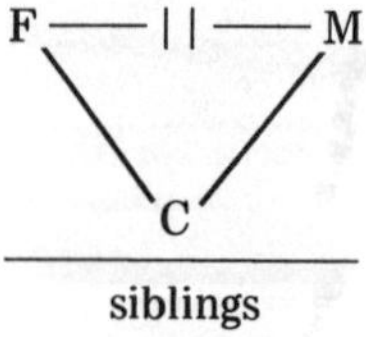

The rigid utilization of one child in spouse conflicts takes several forms. In triangulation, each parent demands that the child side with him against the other parent. Whenever the child sides with one, he is automatically defined as attacking the other. In this highly dysfunctional structure, the child is paralyzed. Every movement he makes is defined by one parent as an attack.

In detouring, another form of the rigid triad, the negotiation of spouse stresses through the child serves to maintain the spouse subsystem in an illusory harmony. The spouses reinforce any deviant behavior in the child because dealing with him allows them to detour or submerge their own spouse subsystem problems in problems of parenting. The parents' detouring may take the form of attacking the child, defining him as the source of family problems because he is bad. In other families, the parents may define the child as sick and weak, then unite to protect him.

The rigid triad can also take the form of a stable coalition. One of the parents joins the child in a rigidly bounded cross-generational coalition against the other parent.

All three types of rigid triad may appear in families with behavioral problems. This triad is the typical transactional pattern, accompanied by other significant family characteristics, in families having children with severe psychosomatic symptoms.

Usually, in such a situation, the therapist's goal is to restructure the subsystem organization according to the paradigm of parent-child functioning (Fig. 32). There are many possible strategies for sub-

Fig. 32

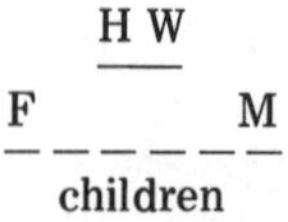

H W
——
F _ _ _ M
children

system restructuring, depending on the individual family's composition, culture, and style. If the child is part of a conflict-avoiding transactional pattern, it may be helpful for the therapist to block him from his usual position in interspouse negotiations. In one case, for instance, where the identified patient is a fifteen-year-old girl suffering from psychogenic vomiting, the therapist takes on the medical responsibility for her symptom. She is not to discuss it with her parents at all. She can talk about it only with him. He thus places himself as a barrier between the girl and her parents, in a maneuver that promotes her autonomy and also promotes closeness between the spouses (Fig. 33).

Fig. 33

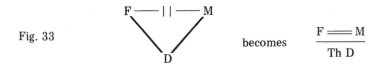

It is possible to pursue the same strategy by using the tactic of increasing the strength of the spouse subsystem boundary without overtly blocking the child from participation. In the case of a sixteen-year-old brittle diabetic girl, the therapist strengthens the parents by rewarding their capacity for nurturance and support. During the initial phase of therapy, he labels their relationship in such positive terms that he increases their affiliation with each other. The husband and wife are then able to negotiate their spouse subsystem problems without the support of their oldest girl, who has always engaged in protective conflict-diffusing interventions. The therapist then moves to affiliate with the excluded girl, thereby furthering the strategy (Fig. 34).

Fig. 34
$$\frac{H = W}{Th = D}$$

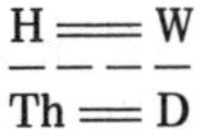

Another possible strategy is to restructure the parents in a coalition against the child who has been a member of the rigid triad. For example, in the Brown family the identified patient, a ten-year-old girl, was referred to treatment because of a life-threatening anorexia nervosa. In a lunch session, the therapist instructs her father to make her eat. The father fails, so the therapist asks the mother, who also fails. Both parents now feel helpless and manipulated by the girl. The therapist offers the interpretation to the family that the girl, who has been treated by the parents as a sick, weak, obedient child, is controlling her parents, putting both of them in a position of helplessness and incompetence in front of the therapist. The parents then join against the girl in a structure that the therapist is able to reinforce as a step toward the therapeutic goal (Fig. 35).

Fig. 35

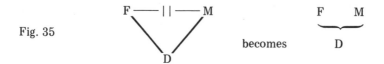

becomes

In a similar case of anorexia in a teenage boy, the family regards the boy's lack of appetite as a reaction to his father's harsh authoritarianism.[2] The mother has joined the boy in a tacit coalition against the father, who feels excluded and guilty. The therapist introduces an adolescent cotherapist, whose function is to help the identified patient move toward his peer world. With the increased distance of the boy from his family comes a movement of the wife toward the husband.

A variety of other strategies can be used in cases of rigid triads. For example, in a family with a phobic boy, the mother's protectiveness of the boy triggers an attack from the father, which increases the mother's protectiveness. The therapist joins the father, making an even stronger attack on the boy and blocking the mother's automatic protective response. This prods the father into a protective stance toward the boy, which increases the affiliation between husband and wife. In another instance, the therapist may use the tactic of increasing the affiliation between an overinvolved parent and child to the point where he unbalances the system. A crisis will develop, forcing the family to develop a new type of response. Another technique is to move another family member into the position of the identified patient, as in the case where the therapist focuses on an older daughter's promiscuity, instead of on the presenting problem of a younger daughter's avoidance of school.

Family transformation does not follow a single therapeutic intervention but requires a continuous involvement in the direction of the therapeutic goal. But many therapists and families spend years meandering in the middle phases of therapy because they have lost the sense of direction that a family map makes explicit. When the complexities of therapy are reduced to the two dimensions of a map, there is some distortion. Nevertheless, structural analysis has the virtue of conveying the sense of therapy as a process directed toward a defined goal.

POSSIBLE PITFALLS OF STRUCTURAL ANALYSIS

The use of structural analysis in determining therapeutic goals and suggesting therapeutic strategies, though effective, has inherent pitfalls. There is the risk of not taking into account the developmental process or all possible family subsystems. There is the further danger of joining and supporting only one subsystem against the others.

Ignoring the Developmental Process. Not to be aware of the family's developmental process and its effect on family structure is a serious pitfall. An example is the therapeutic work with a family composed of the mother, a daughter aged twenty-five, a son aged eighteen, and a daughter aged ten. The father died six years before. The older daughter becomes engaged, and one month later, the younger daughter develops a school phobia and has to be institutionalized in a children's ward. Within three weeks she begins to go to school in the hospital, where she stays for six months. At this point, the son begins struggling with his mother bitterly, and mother and son are taken into family treatment. Each therapist is now working with one subsystem, without considering its relationship to the other subsystems or looking at the developmental process of the entire family.

To consider this family as a system changes the view significantly. It becomes clear that after the husband died, the older daughter joined her mother, forming a system of support by transacting with the mother in an executive subsystem. This structure functions well until the older daughter begins to withdraw from the family, as signified by her engagement. To cope with this forthcoming separation, the mother establishes a strong affiliation with the ten-year-old. The younger daughter responds to the mother's sense of being abandoned by herself withdrawing from the extrafamilial system, remaining at home to reassure her mother.

The removal of the younger child by an agency that is considering only the girl's behavior removes yet another significant source of support from the mother, who is now experiencing her third major loss in six years. She begins to demand more closeness from her son. Strong antagonisms develop from the increased proximity of son and mother, as the son begins to move toward the extrafamilial in the age-appropriate process of separating and gaining individual autonomy. This new problem is in effect iatrogenic, the result of the institution's interventions. The institution has operated in such a way that family stress is increased, instead of working to provide supports to compensate the mother for the imminent loss of her older daughter. If the unit were mother and children, the younger daughter could be rescued from the deviant position, the son would not have to take on the deviant position when the daughter is removed, and the family could be spared a lot of pain.

This blindness to the significance of the complementarity of members in a family system is characteristic of an individual approach to treatment. But a therapist with a systems view can also be subject to it if in his work with one subsystem, he ignores the impact that his interventions will have on the others.

Ignoring Some Family Subsystems. A fourteen-year-old boy becomes withdrawn and begins to act in crazy ways. He has hallucinations and talks to imaginary animals. His parents, a businessman aged forty-six, and a housewife aged forty-two, bring him to a psychiatrist, who diagnoses schizophrenic breakdown. The prognosis is poor, the psychiatrist feeling that the boy's condition will deteriorate further into lifelong chronic schizophrenia. The psychologist at the hospital to which the boy is referred suggests treating the family without hospitalizing the boy. Because the situation seems so hopeless, the psychiatrist and parents agree.

The therapist's assessment of the family is that the spouse subsystem interactions are few and unrewarding. Consequently, the mother and child have an overly close relationship, which keeps the child childish and attached, and excludes the father (Fig. 36).

Fig. 36

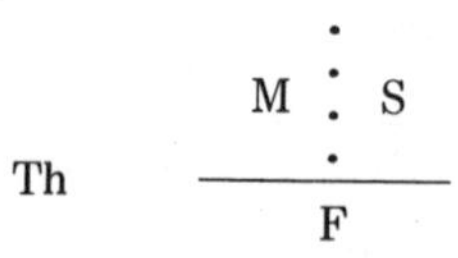

$$\begin{array}{c} \text{M} \vdots \text{S} \\ \text{Th} \quad \overline{} \\ \text{F} \end{array}$$

The therapeutic strategy is to work with the adults so as to increase the husband-wife transactions. When the child participates in family sessions with remarks that are seemingly unrelated to the situation, the therapist does not respond to them. He also suggests to the parents that they refuse to respond to the boy when he makes statements of a psychotic nature. He convinces the parents to go out one night a week without the boy, something they have not done for years (Fig. 37).

Fig. 37
$$\frac{\text{Th} \qquad \text{M} =\!=\!= \text{F}}{\text{S}}$$

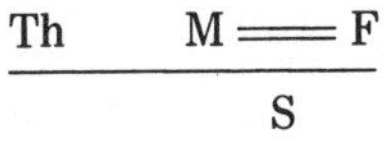

The first time the parents go out alone they come home to find that the boy has slashed his clothing with a razor. The therapist interprets this as the system's response to change. He tells the parents that this is a hopeful sign: they are improving, and their improvement will be manifested by increases in the child's symptoms. The next time they go out, the boy hits a window, breaking it and cutting his wrist, then walks the streets naked. The parents take him to the hospital that night, and the psychiatrist wants to hospitalize him. Again, however, the therapist convinces the parents that this is a response to their increased closeness and is in accordance with the therapeutic plan.

The therapist's assessment of the family dynamics may be correct, but his therapeutic interventions are unnecessarily stressful and possibly dangerous. Treatment of systems in which attention is paid to only one subsystem is frequent. But it is undesirable, uneconomical, and sometimes ethically or humanly incorrect to ignore the other subsystems entirely. In this case, the therapist could have had sessions with the father and son in which the mother was present but not participating. He could have had sessions with the son alone, showing concern for him and including him in therapy. Such an awareness of the child as a suffering individual, instead of as a system member who responds to attempts to restructure with antitherapeutic system-maintaining devices, would have enhanced the total treatment situation without retarding progress toward the goal (Fig. 38).

Fig. 38
$$\text{Th} \qquad \frac{\overset{\text{H W}}{}}{\underset{\text{S}}{\text{F} -\,-\,-\,-\, \text{M}}}$$

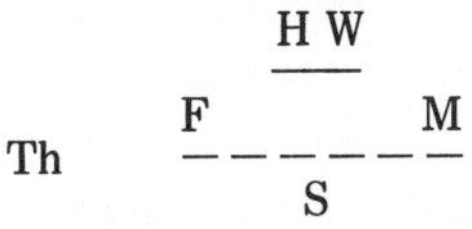

Joining and Supporting Only One Subsystem. Another example of the pitfall of ignoring parts of a system is a family composed of husband, wife, and four children—two boys, aged twenty-one and eighteen, and two girls, aged sixteen and twelve. The oldest boy left home one year ago to join a hippie group. He developed a stable relationship with a girl and became strongly involved in smoking marijuana and experimenting with LSD and speed. He was returned to the family after he and his girlfriend had been hospitalized for toxic psychosis. In the family, he is a strong leader of the sibling subgroup and challenges the authority of his parents, especially the father. The mother sometimes joins the children against the father, complaining about his authoritarian stance.

The therapist, a young single person, feels that the parents, particularly the father, are not allowing the children the autonomy that is necessary and appropriate for adolescents. She sees the children as fighting for freedom from overly rigid parents, and she becomes strongly affiliated to the sibling subgroup. As a result, the father increases his controlling demands and becomes proportionately more ineffective. The wife finds herself caught between her husband, now even more demanding and powerless, and the children, who now have the strong support of the therapist (Fig. 39).

Fig. 39

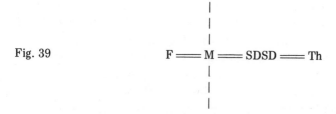

In this case, the introduction of the therapist stresses an already rigid system. The response is for the crystallization and rigidity of transactions to increase. The boundary of the sibling subsystem rigidifies to the point that the parents can no longer exercise their socializing function. If the therapist had supported the parents in their demands for the childrens' respect, she could also have asked the parents to respect the children's rights. By speaking the language of responsibility in the parental subsystem and the language of rights in the sibling subsystem, she could have acted as a bridge between the subsystems (Fig. 40).

Fig. 40

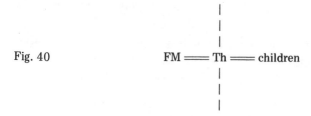

A therapist may join a subsystem in order to see how the system as a whole responds. This is an essential part of the diagnostic process of joining and knowing a family. But maintaining oneself in this position to the point of crystallizing a dysfunctional organization is an act of blindness. This pitfall of structural family therapy can be avoided if the therapist accommodates to the family system to an extent that allows him to experience and assess the stress and pain felt by the family members.

6 The Family in Therapy

What usually brings a family into therapy is the symptoms of one member of the family. He is the identified patient, whom the family labels as "having problems" or "being the problem." But when a family labels one of its members "the patient," the identified patient's symptoms can be assumed to be a system-maintaining or a system-maintained device. The symptom may be an expression of a family dysfunction. Or it may have arisen in the individual family member because of his particular life circumstances and then been supported by the family system. In either case, the family's consensus that one member is the problem indicates that on some level the symptom is being reinforced by the system.

The family, as an open sociocultural system, is continually faced by demands for change. These demands are sparked by biopsychosocial changes in one or more of its members and by various inputs from the social system in which every family is imbedded. A dysfunctional family is a system that has responded to these internal or external demands for change by stereotyping its functioning. Demands for change have been countered by a reification of the family structure. The accustomed transactional patterns have been preserved to the point of rigidity, which blocks any possibility of alternatives. Selecting one person to be the problem is a simple method of maintaining a rigid, inadequate family structure.

The family therapist's function is to help the identified patient and the family by facilitating the transformation of the family system. This process includes three major steps. The therapist joins the family in a position of leadership. He unearths and evaluates the underlying family structure. And he creates circumstances that will allow the transformation of this structure. In actual therapy these steps are inseparable.

As a result of therapy, the family is transformed. Changes are made in the set of expectations that governs its members' behavior. As a result, the extracerebral mind of each family member is altered, and the individual's experience itself changes. This transformation is significant for all family members, but particularly so for the identified patient, who is freed from the deviant position.

In family therapy, the transformation of structure is defined as changes in the position of family members vis-à-vis each other, with a consequent modification of their complementary demands. Although change and transformation are similar terms, in this context they belong to different grammars. In family therapy, transformation, or the restructuring of the family system, leads to change, or the individual's new experience. Transformation usually does not change the composition of the family. The change occurs in the synapses—the way in which the same people relate to each other.

When the therapist joins the family, he assumes the leadership of the therapeutic system. This leadership involves responsibility for what happens. The therapist must assess the family and develop therapeutic goals based on that assessment. And he must intervene in ways that facilitate the transformation of the family system in the direction of those goals. The target of his interventions is the family. Although individuals must not be ignored, the therapist's focus is on enhancing the operation of the family system. The family will be the matrix of the healing and growth of its members. The responsibility for reaching this state, or for failing to do so, belongs to the therapist.

DISEQUILIBRIUM IN TRANSFORMATION

In order to transform the family system, the therapist has to intervene so as to unbalance the system. Jay Haley pointed out the pitfalls of forming a strong affiliation with one member of the family, indicating that if the therapist enters into a coalition with one spouse against the other in a particular session, he should soon repair, and recreate the balance, by coalescing or allying with the other.[1] This kind of balancing technique is helpful in some cases, for the therapist can increase the flexibility of the family and its ability to negotiate conflicts by helping it to attain balance. But in other cases, balancing techniques merely crystallize the rigidity of the family.

For example, a therapist, Ronald Liebman, is working with a rigidly pathogenic family, in which the only daughter, a fourteen-year-old girl with anorexia nervosa, is the identified patient. The therapist's family map reflects an overinvolvement of daughter and mother. The husband and maternal grandmother are joined in a coalition that isolates the mother within the adult subsystem. The mother's only possibility for effectiveness and competence lies in her relationship with her daughter. The therapist's goal is to create distance between the mother and daughter, and to define a boundary around the spouse subsystem that will make it possible to free the girl and the mother from their deviant positions.

The therapist whispers to the girl, "Tell your mother she doesn't love you enough, and that is why you look like a scarecrow." The girl, seeking the therapist's support, obeys. An individually oriented therapist would question this intervention. Because the family therapist is encouraging the girl to be openly aggressive toward her mother, on whom she is pathologically dependent, the individually oriented therapist would worry about the girl's inevitable guilt feelings. He would suspect that she is not expressing her unconscious rage openly but is merely parroting the therapist's words. To blame the mother for the daughter's symptom would seem to him like minimizing the girl's responsibility for her own actions and supporting the mutual dependence of mother and daughter. Finally, he would regard the tactic as unfair to the mother, who is undercut by her husband and her own mother.

The family therapist, however, is by this means taking a step toward the therapeutic goal. The only possibility for improvement in this family lies in the creation of distance between mother and daughter. The therapist's tactics are designed to separate mother and daughter. Accordingly, he forms a coalition with the identified patient against the mother. His intervention skews the balance of all four family members. The mother, deprived of the outlet of her daughter and further stressed by the therapist's criticism, will have no choice but to increase her demands on her husband. The proximity between husband and wife will make it possible to separate the mother and daughter and to free them from their deviant positions.

The structurally oriented therapist may appear to be unfair to individual family members. At any particular transitional moment in therapy, the process will look one-sided. The therapist will seem to be ignoring the complexity of individual dynamics, and may even appear to show insensitivity to the needs of individual family members. However, the total process of therapy will reveal that the therapist is maintaining a sense of contact with the family members in such a way that they follow him even at times when they are experiencing him as unfair. The therapist must be sensitive to the dynamics of the family members, supporting them and confirming some aspects of their personality even when he is disqualifying them in other areas. Any therapist who does not have the capacity to imbue the family with a strong sense of his respect for each one of them as individuals and his firm commitment to healing will lose the family in the processes of transformation.

The family's reliance on the therapist is extremely important in the skewing process. When the therapist unbalances a family system by joining with one member, the other members experience stress. Their response may be to insist on system maintenance. The therapist must counter this by insisting that the family members move in the direction of the therapeutic goals while enduring the uncertainties of the transitional period. This movement is facilitated by the therapist's understanding, support, and confirmation of the family members' experiences and felt needs.

The therapist's use of himself to support family members is particularly crucial in work with pathologically enmeshed families. In all enmeshed families, the processes of differentiation are handicapped. In the pathological range, the family's lack of differentiation makes any separation from the family an act of betrayal. The sense of belonging dominates the experience of being, at the expense of a sense of a separate self. Entering this situation, the therapist works to demarcate psychological and interactional turfs. But if he tries to yank a member of the family system away, he will find that the system pulls more strongly than he can. It is impossible to disengage a member from the system unless he is at the same time engaged at a different level. For example, if a child, as part of a rigid triad, is deeply involved in the affairs of the spouse subsystem and closely allied with one of her parents, one therapeutic goal would be to block the rigid transactional patterns, preventing the use of this child and the reinforcement of her symptoms. One tactic, as well as a goal in itself, would be to return the child to a rewarding position in the sibling subsystem.

Sometimes the interweaving of engagement and disengagement is feasible within the family. For example, while a child is being disengaged from a rigid triad and engaged with the sibling subsystem, the boundary around the spouse subsystem can be strengthened to increase the spouses' engagement. At other times, the therapist may have to use himself as a transitional channel for extrafamilial engagement in order to facilitate the disengagement from the family. Extrafamilial resources can be hooked into the system, as by prodding a mother to find a job that yields satisfactions outside of her family, or introducing as "cotherapist" an adolescent companion to facilitate the movement of a withdrawn adolescent toward the world of his peers.

The therapist must monitor the impact of therapy and of life circumstances on the family and be ready to offer support. Change through therapy, like any other family change, is accompanied by stress, and the therapeutic system must be capable of dealing with it.

The disequilibrium produced by the therapist's entrance into the family and its accommodation to him may be valuable in itself, but may not always be in the direction of the therapeutic goals. The suction of the system may pull the therapist into a contraindicated position. For example, a family comes into therapy because the husband has migraines. He is ashamed of his humble origins, having been the first of his family to go to college. He married a woman whose family he admired for their intellectual accomplishments, and he has great respect for his wife's opinions. She is the rule setter, to whom he accommodates and defers.

The therapeutic goal in this case is to change the relative power positions of the spouses, transforming the family structure so that the man will gain status, securing more respect from his wife and achieving self-respect. To that end, the therapist affiliates with the man in the initial sessions, supporting him and sometimes joining him in a coalition that is critical of the wife.

After four sessions, the wife calls to say that she wants an individual session. She is thinking of having an affair but does not want to hurt her husband by presenting this material in a joint session. When the therapist sees her in the individual session, she lets him know, without making it explicit, that he is the man she wants an affair with. He thinks longingly that as an analyst, he could have interpreted the woman's feeling as a transferential phenomenon, or as resistance to therapy. As a structural family therapist, however, he cannot use this formula. He is faced with two questions. First, how can he help the woman to leave the session without a loss of self-esteem, so as not to handicap therapy? Second, what has he done in previous sessions to downgrade her husband vis-à-vis the therapist, and what can he do to repair that?

The therapist tells the woman to look at an abstract picture on the wall of his office and imagine she is on a date with the man whom she wants as a lover. When she describes her fantasies, he tells her that they are very thin. Her descriptions of the man, he says, are so global and lacking in quality that it is obvious that she would only be exploited in a sexual relationship with him. Indirectly this represents an attack on the woman in several ways. Because she is an actress, she resents having her fantasy description called thin. As an advocate of women's liberation, she reacts strongly to the suggestion that she is seeking a relationship in which she will be exploited. She leaves the office angry and disappointed at the therapist's insensitivity and obtuseness, but ready to continue therapy with her husband. She tells her husband about the session, without telling him that the therapist was her intended lover. During the next session with the couple, the therapist treats the man with great respect, concentrating on his statements and paying close attention to the quality of what he says. He attacks the woman in such a way that the man comes to her defense and attacks the therapist. This helps to correct the skew caused in the previous sessions. Now both spouses have joined in a coalition against the therapist. Within this coalition, they occupy positions of parity. This makes it possible to create a therapeutic system based on the cooperation of peers.

ALTERNATIVE TRANSACTIONS IN TRANSFORMATION

A man separates from his wife, who has manic depressive episodes, when his daughter is six and his son is five. Later he remarries and has another boy. After five years, he brings the two children of his first marriage to live with him and his new family. The family comes into therapy because of his daughter's undue sensitivity, crying spells, and feelings of being unloved.

The second wife, two years older than her husband, has a limited capacity to express feeling. An individually oriented therapist, after watching a session, comments that he would be very concerned about the stepmother's inhibited affective range. He feels that the identified patient, for all her lability, has a great joy of living, which could be potentialized in therapy. The stepmother might dampen this.

The family therapist replies that if he had to search for a stepmother for the daughter of a manic-depressive woman, he would look for a woman with a narrow affective response. In his assessment, the family is suffering from transitional problems. A family of three is being forced to incorporate two new members and become a family of five. The ensuing problems of mutual accommodation and change in structure are what has brought them into therapy.

The father is trying to act as a buffer to protect his wife from his daughter. He enters into power struggles with the daughter, from which the stepmother is excluded. These conflicts escalate without resolution, leaving both father and daughter furious and frustrated. The father, having experienced many similar conflicts with his first wife, tells his daughter that she is too much like her mother. He expresses concern that she too will grow up to be crazy.

The therapist's goal is to free this girl from her mother's "ghost" and to help the family through the processes of transition (Fig. 41).

Fig. 41 $\qquad \dfrac{F D_1}{M D_2} \qquad$ becomes $\qquad \dfrac{F M}{D_1 D_2}$

Accordingly, he follows the strategy of concentrating on the step-mother, eliciting her comments, responding respectfully to her meager inputs, and stating that she is the key to change in the family. This reinforces and increases her activity in the sessions. The therapist forms a coalition with her, saying that her acceptance of the man's children is vital to the family and a meaningful thing for the marriage. But he questions her acceptance of the ghost of the first wife her husband is bringing into their household. The second wife must help her husband exorcise this ghost. The father is attacked for failing to recognize that his daughter is a teenager, not a peer with whom it is appropriate to enter into power struggles. He is also told to realize that she is a person in her own right, not an extension of her mother. The coalition of therapist, wife, and children transforms the family, transitionally making the husband the deviant and freeing the daughter.

This kind of treatment, which focuses on how people can affect and help each other, characterizes the therapist who regards the family as the matrix of healing. The goal is mutual accommodation and support. The stepmother, a wife who has always been afraid to challenge her husband, learns from her young stepdaughter. And while the step-mother is learning from the girl how to challenge, the girl is learning from her stepmother how to retreat.

MOVEMENT IN THERAPY

People's experiences change as their positions relative to one another are transformed. But the question arises as to why family members accept repositioning, and why the transformations are maintained when the therapist is no longer part of the unit. The family comes into therapy asking the therapist only to alleviate the presenting problem. The wonder is that its members then allow and assimilate the therapist's probes, his challenges, and his insistence on change.

Like all therapists, the family therapist challenges people's percep-tions of reality. He conveys to a family member that his experiences are questionable, because the therapist knows that reality is more complex. He erodes each family member's certainty of the validity of his experience. This is not a confrontation technique. Rather, the therapist supports the family members, but suggests that there is something beyond what they have perceived. In effect, he is saying "yes, but . . . " or "yes, and . . . "

He must convince the family members that his "yes, but" or "yes, and" suggestions are derived from their own natures. His position of doubt must be supported by statements that the family members find correct on the basis of their own previous experiences. Although he challenges them on grounds that he can see beyond what they can, he must be able to hook in to alternative possibilities of experience, or alternative codes, already available to family members. What he poses must be a part of the family member's existing repertory.

For example, a wife makes an appointment for therapy because her husband has personal problems and also has great difficulty relating to their two sons. In the first session, the therapist sees the spouses alone. The husband says that he is the member of the family who has the problems. He describes himself as intellectual and logical. Because he is logical, he is sure that he is right; therefore, he tends to be authoritarian.

The therapist interrupts to say that a man who is so concerned with logic and correctness must often be frustrated in life. He criticizes the man for never allowing his wife to perceive the depression he must feel and never allowing her to help him. By this means the therapist is blocking a well-oiled but dysfunctional relationship in terms of an expanded reality. His observation feels right to the man, who acknowledges his depression, and also fits the woman's never-expressed wish for an opportunity to support her husband. Both spouses experience the therapist's challenging, change-requiring input as familiar and welcome, because it recognizes the woman's felt needs and suggests some alternatives that are available to the man. The therapist then assigns a task based on his "yes, but." Under specified circumstances, when the wife feels her husband is wrong, she is nevertheless to side with him against the children.

The parents bring the children to the next session. The adults have performed the assigned task and feel closer. The husband believes that his wife supports him, and she is gratified by the increased sensitivity and decreased authoritarianism he has displayed in response to her support.

When the entire family is seen in therapy, it becomes clear that the children and mother are in a coalition which has isolated the father, making him peripheral and leaving too much of the socialization process to the mother. The children act as a rescue squad. When father sets rules, he does so in a pompous, ex cathedra manner, which makes the mother feel frustrated and helpless. The children begin to misbehave in ways that deflect their father's wrath to them. The younger child is particularly expert at this, and the relationship between him and his father is particularly tense.

The therapist's tactics are to break up the coalition of mother and children, clarifying the boundary around the spouse subsystem and increasing the proximity of husband and wife and of father and children. Accordingly, his strategems must support the father, even though he disagrees with him. He therefore assigns a task that will bring the father and younger son together, excluding the mother. This task also confirms the father in his evident skills of logical thinking and detached observation of behavior, but now directs these skills positively toward a son whom he has always regarded as irritating. The father is to meet with the son at least three times during the week for a period of no longer than one hour. During this period, he is to use his capacity for clear observation and analysis by studying his son, so that during the next session he can describe the son's particular characteristics to the therapist. In this way, the therapist is brought into the contact between father and son as a distant observer. The father, who has always related to this child with impulsive, derogatory, controlling movements, will feel the therapist encouraging him to use his logical skills in relating to his son, inhibiting his impulsiveness. The mother, who has been stressed by her exclusion from this interaction, will nevertheless feel supported in an important area—her wish that her husband become a good father.

The father, mother, and son are all repositioned by the therapist's interventions. Originally they accepted these position changes because the therapist offered them alternatives within their range and held out a promise of more satisfactory arrangements. The family transformation is maintained when the therapist is not there because new dynamics among the family members have been activated by the transformation, and the new transactional patterns are supported by them. The new transactional patterns thus tend toward self-maintenance.

Patients move for three reasons. First, they are challenged in their perception of their reality. Second, they are given alternative possibilities that make sense to them. And third, once they have tried out the alternative transactional patterns, new relationships appear that are self-reinforcing.

THE ROAD IS HOW YOU WALK IT

The concept of transformation deals with large movements in therapy, which take place over time. The therapist must know how to map his goals. But he must also know how to facilitate the small movements that carry the family toward those goals. He must help them in such a way that they are not threatened by major dislocations. A person's ability to move from one circumstance to another depends on the support he receives; he will not move toward the unknown in a situation of danger. Therefore, it is vital to provide systems of support within the family to facilitate the movement from one position to another.

Therapeutic contact occurs on a level of interpersonal immediacy within a specific context. As the poet Jiménez wrote, "the road is not the road, the road is how you walk it." The content of a session is dependent on many idiosyncratic factors, such as the family's own transactional style and the therapist's personality. It is not surprising, therefore, that therapeutic descriptions, seeking to generalize, discuss techniques of treatment in isolation. But therapeutic content relates closely to the current life experience of a family. The family dynamics and structure are conveyed by the content of the communications among its members as well as by the order of those communications.

The content of a session is also influenced by the therapist's input. Two therapists might arrive at basically the same goals and tactics for a family, but the means to those goals would differ markedly because the therapists' styles, as the product of their own life experiences, are different.

For example, my style is partly a product of a childhood spent in an enmeshed family with forty aunts and uncles and roughly two hundred cousins, all of whom formed, to one degree or another, a close family network. My home town in rural Argentina, with only one main street, called "Main Street Number Eleven," had a population of four thousand. My grandparents, two uncles, a cousin, and their families lived on our block. Like an inhabitant of Chinatown, when I walked the street, I felt a hundred cousins were watching me.[2] Thus, I had to learn as a child to feel comfortable in situations of proximity, yet to disengage sufficiently to protect my individuality.

As a young professional, I tended to empathize with children and to blame their parents. After I was married, had children of my own, and was making the mistakes that parents inevitably make, I began to understand parents and to sympathize with them. My life both in Israel, where I worked with Jewish children from many cultural backgrounds, and in the United States, where I worked with black and Puerto Rican families, sensitized me to the universality of human phenomena, as well as to the different ways in which specific cultures prescribe a person's response to these phenomena. I became particularly aware of the manner in which societies coerce their underdogs.

Through the years, I have had a number of successes and made innumerable blunders, which have given me a sense of competence and authority. In my worst moments, this sense of achievement expresses itself in an authoritarian stance, and at other times it allows me to operate as an expert. In the measure to which I have learned to accept myself and to recognize areas in which I will never change, I have developed a sense of respect for the diversity of people's approaches to human problems.

My therapeutic style is organized along two parameters: how to preserve individuation and how to support mutuality. I am always concerned with preserving the boundaries that define individual identity. I do not let one family member talk about others who are present in a session. This rule can be brought alive by telling a family member, "He is taking your voice." I often separate people who are sitting together, and may gesture like a traffic policeman to block interruptions or inappropriate requests for confirmation. I tend to discourage the use of one family member as the repository for others' memories. I approve descriptions of competence and encourage family members to reward any competence that is displayed in a session. I am generous with positive statements about individual characteristics, clothing, a well-turned phrase, or a creative perception. I encourage and join family underdogs, supporting them so that they can win acceptance and change their position. In particular, I support the struggle of growing children for age-appropriate independence. It is often possible to state a problem in this area in terms of comparative ages. "Sometimes you act like a six-year-old, and sometimes you act like a real seventeen-year-old." This formulation becomes a tool for encouraging the development of "seventeen-year-old" behavior.

In encouraging mutuality, my best technique is to display a sense of humor and a general acceptance of the foibles of humans. I tend to challenge the existence of an "I" without a "you." Instead of telling a family member to change, I tell another member, who has a significant complementary relationship with the first, to help the first to change because the first cannot do it alone. This tactic utilizes the power of the family's own system of mutual constraints, which make it difficult for one individual to move without support and complementarity from the others. In effect, I turn other family members into my cotherapists, making of the larger unit the matrix for healing. I avoid making individual interpretations. When a husband is overcontrolling, for example, I may challenge the wife for encouraging her husband's dominance.

I approach family conflicts through sequential interpretations, so that the same pattern is highlighted from different points of view. For instance, in a situation in which a fourteen-year-old child is having difficulties in school and his parents are in conflict about how to deal with this, I might make three interventions. Joining the husband, I would say, "A coalition between your wife and your son is making you helpless." Joining the wife, I would say, "The inability of your husband and son to resolve conflicts is overburdening you, making you responsible for taking care of both of them." Joining the son, I would say, "Your father and mother are arguing about your difficulties in school without giving you any chance to participate. They are keeping you younger than you are." I then ask them to enact a change in the session.

In general, instead of letting people talk about past events, I tend to give situations immediacy by bringing them right into the session. For instance, if I am working with an anorectic patient, I eat with the family. If spouses talk about a conflict, I ask them to enact it. I use space to express proximity and distance, asking people to move about as a way of facilitating or blocking communication and affect.

I have learned to disengage myself and to direct the family members to play out their own drama while I am observing. I am spontaneous with interventions, having learned to trust my responses to families. But I continuously observe the order and rhythm of family communications, making conscious decisions about when to talk to whom.

As a therapist, I tend to act like a distant relative. I like to tell anecdotes about my own experiences and thinking, and to include things I have read or heard that are relevant to the particular family. I try to assimilate the family's language and to build metaphors using the family's language and myths. These methods telescope time, investing an encounter between strangers with the affect of an encounter between old acquaintances. They are accommodation techniques, which are vital to the process of joining.

7 Forming the Therapeutic System

The therapist's methods of creating a therapeutic system and positioning himself as its leader are known as joining operations. These are the underpinnings of therapy. Unless the therapist can join the family and establish a therapeutic system, restructuring cannot occur, and any attempt to achieve the therapeutic goals will fail.

JOINING AND ACCOMMODATION

Joining and accommodation are two ways of describing the same process. Joining is used when emphasizing actions of the therapist aimed directly at relating to family members or the family system. Accommodation is used when the emphasis is on the therapist's adjustments of himself in order to achieve joining. To join a family system, the therapist must accept the family's organization and style and blend with them. He must experience the family's transactional patterns and the strength of those patterns. That is, he should feel a family member's pain at being excluded or scapegoated, and his pleasure at being loved, depended on, or otherwise confirmed within the family. The therapist recognizes the predominance of certain family themes and participates with family members in their exploration. He has to follow their path of communication, discovering which ones are open, which are partly closed, and which are entirely blocked. When he pushes beyond the family thresholds, he will be alerted by the system's counterdeviation mechanisms. The family's impingements on the therapist are the factors that make known the family to him. This process cannot be one-sided: as the therapist accommodates to join the family, the family must also accommodate to join him.

Accommodation operations are not often described in discussions of therapy, being taken as a matter of course. The glue that unites the family and therapist throughout therapy, although acknowledged as necessary, is ignored, while the more dramatic restructuring processes are dealt with. Sometimes the omission is deliberate. Many family therapists prefer not to analyze accommodation techniques on the grounds that they are spontaneous and frequently lie outside the therapist's awareness. They fear that analyzing a therapist's accommodation techniques could inhibit his spontaneity.

For an insight into the accommodation processes, one must turn to anthropology. An anthropologist joins the culture he is studying in order to understand its structure subjectively. In order to do so, according to Claude Lévi-Strauss, the anthropologist accommodates to that culture: "Leaving his country and his home for long periods . . . without mental reservations or ulterior motives, he assumes the modes of life of a strange society. The anthropologist practices total observation, beyond which there is nothing except . . . the complete absorption of the observer by the object of his observations." At the same time, the anthropologist disengages from the society under observation in order to analyze it: "We really can verify that *the same mind which has abandoned itself to the experience and allowed itself to be moulded by it becomes the theatre of mental operations which, without suppressing the experience, nevertheless transform it into a model which releases further mental operations.* In the last analysis, the logical coherence of these mental operations is based on the sincerity and honesty of the person who can say . . . 'I was there.' "[1]

Like the anthropologist, the family therapist joins the culture with which he is dealing. In the same oscillating rhythm, he engages and then disengages. He experiences the pressures of the family system. At the same time, he observes the system, making deductions that enable him to transform his experience into a family map, from which he derives therapeutic goals. To understand and know a family in this intimate, experiential way is a vital component of family therapy.

Although structural maps and the "chess game" approach used here to describe therapy might convey the impression that the therapist manipulates helpless puppets, the reality of family therapy is quite different. Anyone who is engaged in family therapy is constantly impressed by the tremendous difficulty of transforming a family system. The family moves only if the therapist has been able to enter the system in ways that are syntonic to it. He must accommodate to the family, and intervene in a manner that the particular family can accept. Unlike the anthropologist, the therapist is bent on changing the culture he joins, and he has the skills to do so. But his goals, his tactics, and his stratagems are all dependent on the processes of joining.

Over the course of therapy, the therapist's major interventions are designed to move the therapeutic system in the direction of the therapeutic goals. But the therapist must also respond to the immediate elements of each session. These immediate responses may be at variance with the final goals of treatment, because successful restructuring often requires support of the structures that must eventually be challenged. In effect, therapy is measured on two different time scales. The progress of the family toward the therapeutic goals is evaluated as movements over large periods of time. Joining and dealing with immediate problems are evaluated as specific transactions occurring in a single session. Joining techniques may not always advance the family toward the therapeutic goals, but they are successful when they ensure that the family returns for the next session.

Joining a family requires of the therapist a capacity to adapt. Such adaptation, which is here called accommodation, can be either unaware or deliberate. When it is used deliberately, it can speed the early phases of therapy and facilitate treatment.

Maintenance. Maintenance refers to the accommodation technique of providing planned support of the family structure, as the therapist perceives and analyzes it. The system can be maintained on all levels, from the family structure as a whole to the characteristics of the individual members. For example, when Montalvo works with the Gorden family (Chapter 11), he quickly experiences the mother's strong leadership and feels the impact of her insistence that she remain the head of the family and monitor communication with her children. Accordingly, he makes contact with the children through the mother, maintaining the family structure.

The therapist may elect to maintain specific transactional patterns of a family subsystem. When Whitaker talks with Mr. and Mrs. Dodds

(Chapter 10) about the complementarity of their transactions, he supports and highlights their accustomed patterns. For example, he says, "Tell me, Dad, do you resolve her coming up so strong by being easy and quiet?" He reinforces this approach by introducing examples from his personal life: "I married a woman with a lot of fire because I am easy and quiet."

In the Smith family (Chapter 9) the therapist discovers that Mr. Smith expects to monitor contact with his wife. When this rule is broken, Mr. Smith reacts with bizarre behavior, which reinforces a family contract that the therapist is trying to discredit. Consequently, the therapist honors the preferred transactional pattern and makes sure that he has Mr. Smith's permission to contact both Mrs. Smith and their son. Later, when the therapeutic unit is better established, he bypasses this structure so as to diminish the centrality of the identified patient.

Maintenance operations often involve the active confirmation and support of family subsystems. A therapist acknowledges the parents' executive position in a family when he directs his first questions to them, when he respects the family's need to be contacted through the one defined as the central switchboard, or when he temporarily accepts their labeling of the identified patient. When the therapist accepts the spouses' definition of their complementarity, openly enjoys the family's humor, or expresses affection for them, he is using maintenance operations.

The therapist supports family subsystems when he encourages the spouses to support each other in dealing with the adolescent subsystem. He may also support an adolescent subgroup in a large sibling subsystem by recommending that the younger children not come to certain sessions, or by giving them quiet toys to play with while he is talking with the others.

Maintenance operations often involve confirming and supporting an individual's strength and potential, or buttressing a member's position in the family. The therapist may comment on how perceptive a child is in describing a situation, remark on an apt metaphor a family member has used, commend the logic of another person's discussion, or praise the competence with which someone has dealt with a situation. He may compliment a new hairdo or a nice outfit. Every therapist has his own style of confirming individuals. Whitaker is an expert at supporting in such a way as to enhance the possibilities for the expansion of self. Montalvo explores areas of competence and organizes tasks that help family members to achieve skills. Both therapists are generous with their approval.

In the intertwinings of therapy, the maintenance operations may have a restructuring function. When the therapist supports one subsystem, other parts of the family may have to restructure to accommodate to this support. If the therapist supports the weaker spouse, this constitutes a restructuring demand on the stronger spouse. If the parental subsystem is supported, this will have restructuring implications for the sibling subsystem.

Tracking. Tracking is another accommodation technique. The therapist follows the content of the family's communications and behavior and encourages them to continue. He is like a needle tracking grooves in a record. In its simplest form, tracking means to ask clarifying questions, to make approving comments, or to elicit amplification of a point. The therapist does not challenge what is being said. He positions himself as an interested party. Tracking operations are typical of the nonintrusive therapist. The parsimonious "um-hum," the statement prompting continued talk, the repetition of what a person has said, the rewarding of a statement by showing interest, and the question asking for expanded content are time-honored ways by which dynamic and nondirective therapists control the direction and flow of communication.

An action within a session can also be tracked. For example, when Montalvo sees the identified patient in the Gorden family reading, he develops a task in which the girl reads and her mother monitors her competence in reading. Tracking the child's action is thus amplified to include an interpersonal transaction exploring parental functions.

Tracking the content of communications can be useful in exploring the family structure. For example, a therapist working with a highly enmeshed family noted the father's statement that he did not like closed doors. The therapist began to track the door issue. The children, it turned out, were never allowed to close the doors of their rooms. The ten-year-old son had his own room but usually slept in his older sister's room, frequently in the same bed. The spouses' intimacy and sexual life were curtailed because their own door was never closed. Exploring this family's use of its life space and its use of doors became a metaphor for the lack of clear boundaries.[2]

Tracking confirms the family members by eliciting information. The therapist does not initiate an action; he leads by following. He ratifies the family as it is by encouraging and accepting its communications.

Like maintenance, tracking can be used as a restructuring strategy. Ronald Liebman used tracking to create a transitory boundary between the parents of an anorectic girl and the patient. The parents and family met for lunch. The parents, who were extremely involved and anxious, nagged the girl to eat. The therapist, a Jew, encouraged the father, who was an Orthodox Jew, to talk about dietary laws and the rules that supersede the Sabbath law in emergencies. He talked with the mother about the propriety of serving soup as a first course. They discussed the preparation of borscht and whether it should include cabbage as well as beets. It seemed as if the therapist was merely tracking the parents' interests. But while the parents fed the extremely interested therapist with information, the daughter ate her lunch. The therapist had used tracking to position himself as the recipient of the parents' attention, substituting for the daughter, and becoming a boundary between parents and daughter.

Mimesis. Mimesis is a universal human operation. A mother spoon-feeding her baby begins to open her own mouth as he opens his. A person talking to a stutterer slows his speech pattern and may begin to stutter. The long-range effect of mimesis is shown in the tendency for adopted children to look like their adopting parents.

A therapist uses mimesis to accommodate to a family's style and affective range. He adopts the family's tempo of communication, slowing his pace, for example, in a family that is accustomed to long pauses and slow responses. In a jovial family, he becomes jovial and expansive. In a family with a restricted style, his communications become sparse.

The therapist is like the family members in all the universals of the human condition. Therefore, situations will always arise in which they have common experiences. The therapist can emphasize these to blend with the family in a mimetic operation. Communications such as, "I married a woman with fire," "I am a student of the Talmud," "I know what it means to be poor," "I have two adolescent children," and "I had an aunt like that" increase the sense of kinship, indicating that both therapist and family members are, as Harry Stack Sullivan put it, more human than otherwise.

Within the therapeutic system, mimetic operations are usually implicit and spontaneous. In the Dodds family (Chapter 10), Mr. Dodds plays with the baby while the therapist smokes a pipe. When the therapist begins to play with the baby, the father lights his pipe. Experienced therapists perform mimetic operations without even realizing it. Mr. Smith takes off his coat and lights a cigarette. The therapist, who asks him for a cigarette, is aware of performing this as a mimetic operation. But he is unaware of taking off his own coat. As he talks with Mr. Smith, he also scratches his own head in a puzzled, fumbling way, which robs him of authority and increases his kinship with the puzzled, fumbling patient.

Like other processes of accommodation, mimetic operations can be used to restructure. When the therapists affiliate with Mr. Smith and Mr. Dodds by increasing their kinship, the power of the two patients increases.

Accommodation and restructuring processes are intertwined; to separate the two is an artifact of teaching. But only when the accommodation processes, which incorporate the humanity and artistry of the therapeutic encounter, are differentiated can they be studied and taught. Then a therapist can analyze his ability to accommodate, so as to expand his affective range and improve his skills.

DIAGNOSIS

In family therapy, a diagnosis is the working hypothesis that the therapist evolves from his experiences and observations upon joining the family. This type of assessment, with its interpersonal focus, differs radically from the process usually called diagnosis in psychiatric terminology. A psychiatric diagnosis involves gathering data from or about the patient and assigning a label to the complex of information gathered. A family diagnosis, however, involves the therapist's accommodation to the family to form a therapeutic system, followed by his assessment of his experiences of the family's interaction in the present.

The family's approach to their problem is usually oriented to the individual and to the past. The family is brought into therapy by the deviance or pain of one member, the identified patient. Its members' goal is for the therapist to change the identified patient. They want the therapist to change the situation without changing their preferred transactional patterns. In effect, the family is asking for a return to the situation as it was before the symptoms of the identified patient became unmanageable.

The therapist, however, regards the identified patient merely as the family member who is expressing, in the most visible way, a problem affecting the entire system. This does not mean that the identified patient is irrelevant to therapy. He will need special attention. But the whole family must be the target of therapeutic interventions. One aim of the process of diagnosis is to broaden the conceptualization of the problem. The individual focus with which the family has conceptualized and approached the problem must be broadened to include the family's interactions in its current context.

In assessing the family's interactions, the therapist concentrates on six major areas: First, he considers the family structure, its preferred transactional patterns and the alternatives available. Second, he evaluates the system's flexibility and its capacity for elaboration and restructuring, as revealed by the reshuffling of the system's alliances, coalitions, and subsystems in response to changing circumstances.

Third, the therapist examines the family system's resonance, its sensitivity to the individual members' actions. Families fall somewhere on the range between enmeshment, or such extreme sensitivity to individual members' inputs that the threshold for the activation of counterdeviation mechanisms is inappropriately low, and disengagement, or such extremely low sensitivity to individual members' inputs that the threshold for the activation of counterdeviation mechanisms is inappropriately high.

Fourth, the therapist reviews the family life context, analyzing the sources of support and stress in the family's ecology. Fifth, he examines the family's developmental stage and its performance of the tasks appropriate to that stage. And sixth, he explores ways in which the identified patient's symptoms are used for the maintenance of the family's preferred transactional patterns.

Diagnosis in family therapy is achieved through the interactional process of joining. Family structure, the degree of flexibility inherent in it, the system's resonance, and the position of the identified patient are all invisible entities, which can be perceived only through the therapist's accommodation to and probing of the system. The diagnosis of the family appears in the family map. But because this map is intimately related to the idiosyncratic characteristics of both the therapist and family being joined, diagnosis also includes the way in which the family responds to the therapist.

For example, the father of a family is delivering a monolog explaining some aspects of one child's past life that the family considers causal to the child's presenting problem. The therapist listens to this historical material, but he also notes that the father is the family spokesman and that the rest of the family are very quiet. So he probes. Perhaps he asks the mother for her version of what the father is presenting. The family's reaction to this probing is another essential element of the information that the therapist is gathering. Such testing of family organization forms a mini-crisis, which provides valuable data on areas of flexibility and the limits of tolerance.

The content of a family's communications to a therapist, particularly in the beginning, is usually carefully organized and has often been rigidified by frequent rehearsal. It is an official version of events, which yields minimal information to the therapist. The material that the therapist elicits when he joins the family is under less cognitive control and is usually less guarded, giving a glimpse of the underlying transactional patterns.

In a sense, an interactional diagnosis is achieved by the process of gathering different classes of information. What people say, organized into a logical sequence in terms of the significance of the material presented, is important. So are nonverbal cues, such as the pitch of the voice or frequent hesitations. Additional material can be gleaned from the order of remarks: who speaks to whom and when. Then the therapist's prodding yields information about alternative transactional patterns, indicating the flexibility of the family organization when it is mobilized in the context of the therapeutic session.

The therapist's impact on the family is part of a family diagnosis. The therapist's entrance is in itself a massive intervention. The family therapist must recognize his influence on the picture being presented by the family. He cannot observe the family and make a diagnosis from "outside."

Interactional diagnosis constantly changes as the family assimilates the therapist, accommodates to him, and restructures, or resists restructuring interventions. That is another difference between this type of diagnosis and the standard psychiatric diagnosis. An individual diagnosis is a static label, which emphasizes the individual's most salient psychological characteristics and implies that these are resistant to changes in social context. In family therapy, individuals and families are seen as relating and changing in accordance with their social context. The advantage of an evolving diagnosis related to context is that it provides openings for therapeutic intervention. Diagnosis and therapy become inseparable.

This type of diagnosis is also inseparable from prognosis. The enactment of family transactions after the family has joined the therapist reveals alternative transactional patterns which can be identified as significant in therapeutic growth. Any type of diagnosis is merely a way of arranging data. The family therapist has the advantage of working with the concept of a system of interconnected people who influence each other. Therefore, if his arrangement of data leads him to an insoluable problem, he searches for a different angle on the same complex phenomena. For example, the diagnosis of Mr. Smith as an agitated, depressed individual gives the psychiatrists treating him limited directions for therapy and a poor prognosis. The family therapist's first, transitory diagnosis for Mr. and Mrs. Smith as an interacting couple is that Mrs. Smith is in need of Mr. Smith's help in overcoming her sexual problem. This diagnosis is both as correct and as partial as the previous one, but it has the advantage of leading to a completely different treatment procedure, which helps the Smith family.

THE THERAPEUTIC CONTRACT

An essential element of the formation of a therapeutic system is the agreement on a therapeutic contract. The family wants the presenting problem solved without interference with their preferred transactional patterns. But change in the identified patient will probably depend on family transformation. The family therapist broadens the focus of the problem to include family interactions, and in most cases some aspects of the family interactions will become targets of the therapy. Consequently, the family and the therapist must come to an agreement on the nature of the problem and on the goals for change. This contract may not have a very clearly defined nature, but it must be present. At first it can, if necessary, be very limited, but it will expand or change with time. Like the diagnosis, it evolves as therapy progresses.

The contract holds out a promise of help for the family with the problem that has brought it into therapy. If broadening the focus is not at first possible, the contract may be confined to the index problem: "I will help you with Joe." Soon, however, its coverage will expand: "You have a problem in disciplining your children; I will help you with this problem too." Finally, the contract can cover an entirely new area: "You and your spouse are on opposite sides in relation to child rearing. We will need to explore this area together."

The therapeutic contract also specifies the logistics of therapy. The treatment may be conducted in the office, in the home, at school, or it may shift from place to place. The therapist may be restricted to dealing with intrafamilial problems, or he may help the family in difficulties with other agencies. The therapeutic contract specifies how frequently sessions will be scheduled, and for how long. All of its terms can change as therapy evolves, but some degree of understanding must be reached at the start.

JOINING SUBSYSTEMS

In general, joining a subsystem constitutes a restructuring intervention, because other family members must regroup to absorb the impact of the alliance of the powerful therapist with another subsystem. However, the technique also depends on the therapist's skill at accommodation and confirmation.

When the therapist works with a family, he joins the various subsystems differently, accommodating to each one's internal transactional patterns, to its style, affect, and language. For example, the language, needs, and feelings of adolescent children are very different from those of younger children. The themes and affect of the parental subsystem can change dramatically when the parents meet with the therapist separate from the children. A therapist's accommodation techniques must take into account all the different styles and types of thinking that appear in different subsystems in different contexts.

One therapeutic skill that is often neglected is the accommodation to children. Some family therapists tend to accommodate to the adults in the family, to the detriment of the children. This skew may sometimes be justified because the parents have more power and are more apt to be the natural instruments for family restructuring. But at other times the reason for this approach seems to be the therapist's own lack of skill in accommodating to children at different stages of development.

A young child often responds to abstract questions asked by a stranger with "I don't know" or a monosyllabic answer. He may look at his parents, expecting them to answer for him or at least to give a nonverbal cue on how to answer. This may be because the child is responding defensively, but it may also be because the question was couched in "adult language" or was too abstract, making it inappropriate to the child's level of cognitive development.

A family therapist must be able to accommodate to children's talk. In the Dodds family session, the therapist's most powerful joining operation comes when he is trying to make contact with the ten-month old baby. He sits on the floor and tickles him. The mood of the family changes, and the blaming mother of the soiling identified patient becomes the proud mother of the active, happy infant. There is a visible increase in the sense of acceptance and support among family members. In the Gorden family, when the therapist first makes contact with a frightened, scapegoated child, he uses the concrete language of gestures. "Was the fire this big," he gestures, "or this big?" To win responses from this anxious child, he continues by asking questions that require only a "yes" or "no." When Mandy has answered three or four times the therapist ventures to ask a question that requires a description. He gradually increases the complexity of his language. With the parental child, he uses body contact and bantering as a way of driving home his restructuring message that the parental child should leave more of the mothering to the mother. "You are busy, man," he tells him, and "you are overemployed."

Using different family subsystems can be a useful technique. Some family therapists suggest that treatment should be conducted with all family members present, so as to ensure open communications. Working only in the presence of all family members would certainly inhibit the development of family secrets and ghosts, but there are circumstances in which working with separate subsystems is a powerful restructuring device. In the highly enmeshed family, for instance, the weakness of the boundaries of a high resonance system is pathogenic. In the family with open doors, restructuring was based on the defining of clear boundaries around husband and wife and around the teenaged daughter, which allowed a degree of privacy to both subsystems.

In a family in which the spouses continually attack each other in escalating conflicts, which plateau only when the parents unite in blaming one of their adolescent children, the therapist was able to deflect this dysfunctional pattern by having the parents bring only the three children under six. For three sessions, therapist, parents, and children sat on the floor building towers and racing cars. Among the youngsters, it was possible to introduce a sense of support between the parents that was impossible with the previous grouping.

When therapy begins, the therapist invites all the members of a household to the sessions. If he knows it to be an extended family, he includes the grandparents. If there is another adult significantly involved with a single-parent family, he tries to make contact with that person. He asks the family to bring all the children, including the youngest, to the initial sessions. His observations of the total family help the therapist identify the different ways in which different family members participate in the maintenance of dysfunctional transactional patterns. It also gives clues as to the relative power of different family members to effect or resist changes in the family. Armed with these observations, the therapist can strategically contact certain family subsystems, excluding others.

Including and excluding family members in the current therapeutic unit is a powerful strategy for exploring how subsystems function in changing contexts. A parental child may be obedient while his parents are present and turn into a despot when he is in charge of the sibling subsystem. A mother who is competent with her children can become ineffective in the presence of her own mother. A child who is protected by his mother may be scapegoated in the sibling subsystem. In families with many children, the sibling subsystem becomes further subdivided. Meeting the parents and the different sibling subgroups presents very different views of family transactional patterns.

With some families, the therapist always works with the total group. In others, he selects the group that he feels is most appropriate, alternating different groupings depending on the developing dynamics. In general, the therapist should protect the spouses' privacy from intrusion. When working with families with adolescent children, the therapist can hold individual sessions with each adolescent, which allows for exploring issues autonomously and for establishing a relationship with a significant extrafamilial adult that would not be possible within the total family group.

Working with different segments of the family can be a restructuring technique. For example, the therapist can divide members of a coalition. He can see two family members who have been in a stable coalition for some sessions without the member whom they have been opposing, thereby developing a relationship that does not require a coalition against someone. Opposing members can be seen together to alter their pattern of transactions. For instance, the therapist assigns the Gorden mother the task of teaching the child she has been scapegoating how to be competent in lighting matches. In the session, while all family members are present, he establishes a boundary that keeps the other three children from interfering in the development of a pleasurable mother-patient transaction.

Sometimes the activity of an inappropriately central member of the family can be curtailed within a session. The therapist can block his input by stepping up his own activity. He can send the central member out to watch the session from behind a one-way mirror. Or he can simply increase the distance between this member and the rest of the family by changing the seating so as to limit his participation. Then processes that would otherwise have remained submerged may appear.

The therapist can act as a family boundary maker by joining with one subsystem of the family and excluding others during sessions of the entire family. He may, for instance, create geographical turfs that facilitate communication only between certain members of the family. All these subsystem interventions are also valuable as probes in the process of diagnosis.

JOINING AND RESTRUCTURING

The separation of joining and restructuring is an artificial distinction, which does not characterize the natural unfolding of therapy. The therapeutic unit is in continual movement, and the processes of joining, probing, observing, helping, making a therapeutic contract, and sparking transformation occur again and again in kaleidoscopic sequence. For example, developing a family diagnosis is part of the process of joining. But it is quite possible that in actual therapy a restructuring intervention may develop before a tentative diagnosis has been made.

The interweaving of accommodation and restructuring is both interesting and complex. It is even possible to group family therapists according to their avowed use of accommodating and restructuring operations. In the "transferential" group, the therapist is not thought of as joining the family. The processes of accommodation are considered as an incidental part of therapy, to be controlled only if they become countertransferential. The process of family restructuring is seen as occurring as a result of the therapist's interpretations—his input into the family from a disengaged position. The therapist is outside, looking in.

In the "existential" group, the therapist and family are regarded as accommodating to each other. Change in the family is believed to occur as a result of this mutual accommodation, and growth is therefore expected to be unspecific and generic. Restructuring operations and strategies are dismissed as manipulative and growth inhibiting. The therapist operates from within, without disengaging.

In the "structural" approach both types of operation are considered essential for therapy. The accommodation processes are specific operations, by which the therapist gains subjective knowledge of family transactional patterns and positions himself as the leader of the therapeutic system. The restructuring operations, which may include tasks to be carried out at home away from the therapist, demand specific changes in family organization. The therapist alternates from the position of engagement typical of the existential approach to the disengaged position of the expert. All these schools, however, represent a theoretical stance more than they describe a therapist's actual behavior. Such behavior may differ greatly from the therapist's avowed theoretical position.

8 Restructuring the Family

Restructuring operations are the therapeutic interventions that confront and challenge a family in the attempt to force a therapeutic change. They are distinguished from joining operations by the challenge they pose. Joining operations do not challenge; they decrease the distance between family and therapist, helping the therapist to blend with the family as together they participate in the events of the therapeutic session.

Restructuring operations and joining operations are nevertheless interdependent. Therapy cannot be performed without joining, but it will not be successful without restructuring. Often it is difficult to distinguish between the two. Joining can be used as a restructuring technique. But when a joining operation is used to restructure, it does so without confronting the family. The technique can be compared to jujitsu. An expert in jujitsu uses his opponent's own movement to throw him off balance. In using joining operations to restructure, the therapist uses the family's own movement to propel it in the direction of the therapeutic goals.

In joining operations, the therapist becomes an actor in the family play. In restructuring, he functions like the director as well as an actor. He creates scenarios, choreographs, highlights themes, and leads family members to improvise within the constraints of the family drama. But he also uses himself, entering into alliances and coalitions, creating, strengthening, or weakening boundaries, and opposing or

138

supporting transactional patterns. He uses his position of leadership within the therapeutic system to pose challenges to which the family has to accommodate.

Restructuring operations are the highlights of therapy. They are the dramatic interventions that create movement toward the therapeutic goals. But they depend for their success on a therapeutic unit that is firmly established. When the therapeutic unit is solidly formed, restructuring operations must be designed to allow for periods of consolidation and regrouping as the family changes.

When the therapist joins the family, he has two main tasks. He must accommodate to the family, but he must also maintain himself in a position of leadership within the therapeutic unit. He must resist being sucked into the family system. He must adapt himself sufficiently to the family organization to be able to enter it, but he must also maintain the freedom to make interventions that challenge the family organization, forcing its members to accommodate to him in ways that will facilitate movement toward the therapeutic goals.

If a therapist succumbs to the family's pressure to join it in ways that supplement and perpetuate the family organization, he may lose his freedom of action. He then becomes powerless to impose restructuring interventions. His input only complements a dysfunctional system and helps to crystallize the maladaptive transactional patterns he should be working to restructure. For example, a family comes into therapy because the mother cannot control her active preadolescent children. The therapist finds it impossible to conduct a session in the midst of the family's chaotic activity, so he begins to impose controls on the children, taking over the functions of parenting within the family. By complementing instead of working to restructure, he is sucked into the family system. The mother entirely relinquishes her tenuous hold on the children, becoming dependent on the therapist to such an extent that he has to continue performing parental and other executive functions for his "adopted" family in order to keep it going.

The therapist can maintain his therapeutic maneuverability and his freedom to manipulate himself as well as the family only from a position of leadership. The word "manipulation" sometimes causes problems when applied to therapy because of its negative connotations. Yet families come into therapy because they are in pain and need help. Families with chronic dysfunctional patterns can be helped only by changing those patterns. The pain can be reduced only when the family's functioning improves. The therapist's job is to manipulate the family system toward planned change. He must be able to engage with the family in operations that facilitate movement. The therapeutic contract must recognize the therapist's position as an expert in experimental social manipulation.

There are at least seven categories of restructuring operations: actualizing family transactional patterns, marking boundaries, escalating stress, assigning tasks, utilizing symptoms, manipulating mood, and supporting, educating, or guiding. This list is by no means exhaustive, and it fails to cover the many variations governed by the individual styles of therapists and their client families. Every therapist prefers some techniques over others, and uses them in different ways according to his own personality and resources and those of each family he treats.

ACTUALIZING FAMILY TRANSACTIONAL PATTERNS

Although the therapist must maintain his position of leadership, he must avoid the danger of this position, namely, the risk of becoming overcentralized. A family comes into therapy looking for help from an expert. They expect to explain themselves to him and be advised by him. Therefore, they tend to address themselves solely to him, describing the situation as they see it.

If the therapist does not check this tendency, the session may become programmed in such a way that he remains central, even when he is silent. Everything may be directed toward him and modified accordingly. He may find himself constantly participating in successive dyads, unable to disengage in order to observe. As a result, the session may be directed according to the therapist's own assumptions and hunches. Or it may follow the lines laid down by the family member who is most active in the context of the therapeutic session. The transactions thus elicited may be very different from the family's normal transactions.

Another danger lies in allowing the session to be confined to a family's descriptions, because a family's real transactional patterns may be entirely outside their awareness. They may scrupulously describe how they think they relate to each other, without realizing that their transactional patterns are in fact quite different. In order to get a true picture, the therapist must move beyond the family's verbal self-description.

Accordingly, the therapist watches for noverbal clues that confirm or contradict what the family is telling him. A communication is always reinforced, qualified, or denied by the interpersonal context of the transaction. The Smith family is a good example of this multiple-level presentation of data. Mrs. Smith complains that her husband is a silent person. But she consistently interrupts and silences him when he starts to talk. She says that her husband is a person she respects and even fears. But her minute descriptions of his need to control her are clearly disrespectful of a man she really perceives as sick and weak. She says that her husband controls the couple's contact with the extrafamilial world. But her tenacity and the force of her monologs leave her clearly in control of their contact with the therapist.

The therapist, as he listens to what Mrs. Smith is saying, simultaneously registers the processes that are outside the couple's awareness. He gathers the rehearsed material, in which both spouses present Mr. Smith as the problem, but he also experiences and evaluates the transactional patterns that are reinforcing Mr. Smith's symptoms. This synergistic skill yields a complexity of data that would otherwise be unobtainable.

Enacting Transactional Patterns. There is considerable value in making the family enact instead of describe. The therapist can gather only limited data from the family's descriptions. To amplify his data, he must help them transact, in his presence, some of the ways in which they naturally resolve conflicts, support each other, enter into alliances and coalitions, or diffuse stress.

His presence is always a modifying factor. He can nevertheless create family scenarios by directing certain family members to interact with each other in a clearly delineated framework. The instructions must be explicit, such as, "Talk with your father about that." This kind of scenario minimizes the tendency to centralize the therapist and helps the family members to experience their own transactions with a heightened awareness. From the therapist's point of view, it also helps him see the family members in action. Only then can he begin to understand the family structure that underlies the idiosyncratic behavior of its members.

Recreating Communication Channels. It is relatively easy to actualize dialogs. The therapist can listen for a situation in which a family member is talking about the behavior of another member, and direct the speaker to talk with the other member, instead of about him. This process, however, may be blocked by a family that insists on using the therapist as a listener. The members may openly object that they have discussed the problem among themselves many times and now want to talk to the therapist about it. Or they may begin to talk to each other and quickly return to the therapist. The therapist, therefore, must have a number of techniques for encouraging intrafamilial communication in the session. He may insist that people talk with each other. He may avoid looking at anybody, focusing his gaze on an object. He may move his chair back. He may refuse to respond when addressed, simply indicating another family member with a gesture. He may even leave the room, to observe the family from behind a one-way mirror. After he has used these techniques a number of times, the family members will accept having to talk to each other as a rule of the therapeutic system.

Now a new vista opens for the therapist. He can begin to pay less attention to the logic of content and more attention to the patterned sequences in which family transactions occur. His observations may serve merely to gather data that will later suggest a focus for intervention. Or they may become the focus for immediate therapeutic interventions. In the Smith family, watching the couple interact makes the therapist realize that he cannot be successful in creating a dialog unless he takes a strong position of leadership supporting Mr. Smith. He therefore joins the husband in a coalition against his wife, using this technique to organize Mr. Smith's participation in such a way that he appears more competent.

Manipulating Space. Geographical rearrangement is another technique for enacting the family descriptions. Location can be a metaphor for closeness or distance between people. In the Gorden family, the boundary around the parental subsystem (mother and oldest son) has become impermeable to the scapegoated child, Mandy. The therapist changes seats with the mother so that she is sitting next to her scapegoated daughter while they explore an issue. The therapist sits next to the parental child, so as to block the boy's interference with the mother-daughter transaction (Fig. 42). The therapist thus

	M			
	| | | |			
Fig. 42	S		M	Th
	———	becomes	| | | |	
	D		D | S	

rearranges four people to indicate a therapeutic goal: mother transacting with daughter without interference from son.

When a family comes in for the first session, the way in which they position themselves can provide clues to alliances and coalitions, centrality, and isolation. If a child moves quickly to sit in the chair next to his mother's and moves his chair close to hers, the therapist can make an assumption about this dyad. Later, he may notice that the child looks at his mother before answering a question. If he wants to block this sequence, or to indicate that increasing distance between the child and his mother will be a therapeutic goal, he can do so by separating them and positioning the child so that he cannot catch his mother's eye.

In the Dodds family, the index patient sits away from the rest of his family, on the other side of the cotherapist. The senior therapist asks the cotherapist to change seats with the patient's younger brother, seating the boys together, so that the index patient is supported and placed back inside the family. Later, the senior therapist sits on the floor to play with the baby, using this position to facilitate the enactment of nurturing and supporting fantasies in the family.

Positioning can also be a technique for encouraging dialog. In the Smith family, the therapist asks Mr. Smith to look at his wife and talk to her. When Mr. Smith moves his chair away from his wife, the therapist moves next to Mr. Smith and moves Mr. Smith's chair nearer to his wife's. Mr. Smith then puts a wastepaper basket between him and the therapist. All the drama of a fear of closeness is acted out in these simple moves.

Positioning can be an effective way of working with boundaries. If the therapist wants to create or strengthen a boundary, he can bring members of a subsystem to the center of the room and have other family members move their chairs back so that they can observe but cannot interrupt. If he wants to block contact between two members, he can separate them, or he can position himself between them and act as go-between. Spatial manipulation has the power of simplicity. Its graphic eloquence highlights the therapist's message.

MARKING BOUNDARIES

For healthy functioning, a family must protect the integrity of the total system and the functional autonomy of its parts. Each family member and each family subsystem must negotiate the autonomy and interdependence of its psychodynamic turf.

The family therapist tries to help the family create the flexible interchange between autonomy and interdependency that will best promote the psychosocial growth of its members. Independence per se is not the goal. The derogatory connotation of the notion of dependence in individual psychodynamic theory is not carried over into family therapy, which recognizes the interdependence of all systems. The goal is to attain the correct degree of permeability of boundaries.

In an enmeshed family, the boundaries must be strengthened to facilitate the individuation of family members. The therapist joins an enmeshed family with an eye toward increasing the clarity of boundaries. In families toward the disengaged end of the enmeshment-disengagement continuum, he moves to decrease the rigidity of boundaries, facilitating the flow among subsystems in ways that allow an increase in the family's supportive and governing functions.

Delineating Individual Boundaries. Individual autonomy can be protected and promoted by simple rules that are imposed as part of the overall rules governing the therapeutic unit. For instance, the therapist and family should listen to what a family member says and acknowledge his communication. The family members should talk to each other, not about each other. Family members should not answer a question directed to another, talk about other members while they are present, or require one member to act as the memory bank for all the family.

It is not difficult to impose these rules within the session. If one family member begins to answer a question directed to another, the therapist can silence the speaker with a gesture and, if necessary, say something like, "Joe, that question was directed toward you." In general, I tend to inhibit any communication from one family member that describes another's actions or feelings. This can be done gently, saying, "He was there and you were not, so maybe he could describe it." Or blocking such communication can be done harshly, confronting the family member with his intrusion.

Children in a family should be differentiated, receiving individual rights and privileges according to their age and position in the family. The therapist can explore the family's own differentiation, using questions such as, "Who chose the clothes of the eight-year-old?" "What is his bedtime?" "What are the family rules for eating, watching television, taking baths?" The therapist can also watch how a child answers questions directed at him. Some children respond autonomously; others look at one parent before answering or refer the question to the parent.

If the children's individual autonomy seems to be hampered within a family, the therapist should help the family underline differences among the children, emphasize their right to differences, and help the parents make specific demands and rewards according to each child's developmental stage. For example, in the family that forbade closed doors, a highly enmeshed system, the therapist's approach was to assign a task appropriate to the older daughter's developmental stage. She was to close the door of her bedroom. He told the younger daughter that she should do the same when she was older.[1]

Subsystem Boundaries. Spouse subsystem boundaries should be clear enough to protect the couple from intrusion by children or by adult members of the extended family. Family therapists must often work in this area, because an inappropriate rigidity or diffusion of the spouse subsystem boundary is a common source of dysfunctional transactional patterns. Sometimes it is helpful to assign tasks that encourage spouse subunit transactions. For example, in the family with open doors, the therapist tells the parents to evict the children from their bedroom for one hour each evening. The parents are to spend this hour in their bedroom alone, with the door closed. In the case of the Smiths, the therapist asks the grandfather and son to leave the room before he begins to discuss sexual matters with the couple.

In addition, the family must have an executive subsystem that can make decisions, particularly with regard to child rearing. Usually the parents form this subsystem. The parental subsystem must have authority. A child must be able to experiment with growing up, knowing that the parental subsystem will set the limits of the permissible. A therapist must therefore intervene in a family in ways that support the differentiated allocation of power. For example, a son who is well inducted into the family's formulation that all problems stem from his father's intrapsychic illness criticizes his father with impunity. The therapist expresses anger at this, indicating that the boy should show respect for his father.

The sibling subsystem also needs a protective boundary so that it can exercise its functions of offering children the opportunity to learn cooperation, competition, ways of avoiding or surrendering, how to gain or lose an ally, and other skills of living with peers. Parents must respect this opportunity for growing without their help or interference.

In the Brown family (Chapter 12) the sibling subsystem's support and reinforcement of a nine-year-old girl's anorexia nervosa is just as

significant as is the reinforcement from the spouse subsystem. Therefore, the therapist develops tasks for the sibling subsystem, and the
parents are specifically excluded from intervening. He uses the
technique of bringing the children into the center of the room to
negotiate or explore issues. He remains with the parents on the
periphery, helping them to observe without participating, teaching
them to respect their children's autonomy.

The rigid triad poses special challenges in boundary drawing. When a
cross-generational transactional pattern, usually involving the parents
and one child, becomes encased in a rigid boundary, it generates
dysfunctional transactional patterns. The therapist must work to
redraw the boundaries: strengthening the spouse subsystem boundary
so the spouses can negotiate spouse issues without involving a third
member, strengthening the boundary that protects the third member's
autonomy, and weakening the boundary surrounding the rigid triad so
that the subsystem becomes more open.

When the boundaries around a subsystem are strengthened, the
functioning of that subsystem will increase. Processes that could not
occur when other family members intruded will now appear. This is
clear in the Gorden family. The therapist delineates two subsystems.
He has the mother work alone with the child she has been scapegoating, strengthening the boundary around this dyad, which has been
too weak. He puts the parental child in charge of the other children,
weakening the boundary around the parental subsystem, which has
excluded the scapegoated child. Within this boundary system, the
mother is able to work with the scapegoat in a competent, nurturant
fashion.

In some families, sharper separations are necessary or helpful. A
system can become more conflictual as the number of its members
increases. Changes in the number of members in a system can
themselves cause a significant transformation of the system. Sometimes the removal of the symptom bearer results only in the displacement of an unresolved conflict to another symptom bearer. But at
other times changes can occur simply in the process of separating one
family member from the family. Short periods of hospitalization of
one family member during an acute period of family stress can be not
only a necessary palliative but also an essential part of the process of
changing the family as a system.

The therapist can impose boundaries by working selectively with
different subsystems of a family. He starts work by seeing all the

members of a nuclear family, but as he derives a family map, he may spot an area in which it would be useful to increase or decrease the membership of the therapeutic unit. Some therapists prefer to work only with the spouses or parents. Others prefer to work with as much of a family's social network as can be mustered. Still others prefer to work with multiple families.

I prefer to work with the nuclear family, sometimes changing the group composition. When working with adolescents, I always include individual sessions with the adolescent children. When working with large families, I work with the subsystems—parents alone, parents with older children, parents with younger children, the sibling subsystem. In some families, working with significant members of the extended family is important. Sometimes parents may select the members who will participate in a session. With other families, the selection of subgroups is determined by restructuring dynamics. The therapist can join with an isolated father and his children, excluding the mother, to allow new functions to develop. A dominating parent can be sent behind a one-way mirror, so that he can participate without being able to control. Young children can be brought in to a session to provide a lessening of conflict. The therapist always works with his map of the total family in mind. Even when he is working intensively with a subgroup, his goal is the total restructuring of the family.

ESCALATING STRESS

Families coming for treatment have usually developed dysfunctional transactional patterns for handling stress. The identified patient is at the center of these patterns. The family is frequently stuck, unable to experiment with alternative ways of relating. The therapist who joins them in the therapeutic system must explore whatever alternative behaviors the family organization can permit. He must experience and probe both the flexibility of the family system and its capacity to restructure and grow with his help.

The therapist's skill at producing stresses in different parts of the family system will give him, and sometimes the family members themselves, an inkling of the family's capability to restructure when circumstances change. His input and his expert prodding produce new contexts, or changed circumstances, to which the family must adapt under his eye.

Blocking Transactional Patterns. The simplest maneuver that the therapist can use to produce stress is to dam the flow of communication along its usual channels. For example, in the Gorden family, the parental child enters in his usual role of translating the mother's communications to the other children, and theirs to her. The therapist intervenes, saying "Excuse me, Morris" and "Go ahead," to the interrupted child. Blocking the parental child's intervention allows an increased contact between the mother and the other children, who have been separated by Morris' interference. Five minutes later in the session, the flexibility of the family organization is manifested. When Morris again tries to help his mother understand his sister, the mother, imitating the therapist, tells him not to interrupt.

Emphasizing Differences. A therapist can produce stress by highlighting differences that the family has been glossing over. He is attuned to the ways in which family members qualify each others' statements, "improve" a family member's message, or simply disagree. He may listen to one member's opinion on an issue, then turn to another member and say, "What is *your* opinion?" Or he can make his intervention even more specific, saying, for instance, "It seems that you and your wife don't see eye to eye on this issue; can you discuss it?"

Developing Implicit Conflict. A family's methods for defusing conflict operate swiftly and automatically. A husband may attack himself whenever he thinks his wife is about to attack him, taking the wind out of her sails and styling himself a weak man, who should therefore be protected. He abandons any position of strength because the spouse subsystem does not allow a confrontation that would force the appearance of hidden conflict. A child can become disruptive or display other symptoms if his parents begin to enter conflict. In the first case, the therapist acts like the classic "helper," offering to hold the opponents' jackets. Perceiving that the husband is using self-derogation as a technique for avoiding contact, and hence conflict, with his wife, the therapist forces the couple to make contact. In the second case, the therapist works to destroy the dysfunctional conflict-detouring mechanism by breaking up the rigid triad, blocking the child's interference in parental conflict.

Joining in Alliance or Coalition. The therapist can produce stress by temporarily joining one family member or subsystem. This type of entrance into the family structure requires careful planning and an ability to disengage, so that the therapist is not sucked into the family war.

He may join different family members serially. In this case, he would ally with one member and fight on his side, then shift, distributing his favors fairly and developing successive stresses in different parts of the family system. For example, a therapist working with a highly enmeshed family sides with the father to help him state his grievances against his wife, then with the wife to help her state her grievances against the father, and then successively with each of the children, as the family works to develop differentiated rules and appropriate supportive responses.

The therapist must also know when and how to join with one family member for a longer period. This approach is especially necessary with families that rigidly deny or defuse conflict and with families that persistently refuse to accept the idea that the family as a whole is the problem. These rigid systems can be jarred into motion by joining with one family member, usually a parent, for a long time, such as four or five sessions. If the therapist joins one spouse against the other for a long period, he stresses both spouses. The impact challenges the spouse subsystem's threshold of stress, its accustomed ways of transacting, and its preferred methods of negotiating or avoiding conflict.

For example, in one family, conflict in the spouse subsystem is avoided by scapegoating a son. When the wife challenges her husband for not making more money, he directs his attention to the boy, correcting his behavior and thereby re-establishing his own threatened sense of competence. When the husband challenges the wife for being a sloppy housekeeper, she begins to talk about the child's misbehavior in school. The therapist joins the husband in a coalition against the wife, strongly supporting his demand for more order in the house. This technique results immediately in the emergence of spouse conflict which, with the therapist's help, is negotiated within the spouse subsystem, freeing the boy.

When the therapist joins one family member, he must be acutely aware of his ally's threshold of endurance and of the other family members' threshold of endurance. He runs a strong risk of alienating the target of the coalition and, frequently, the whole family. Even in the midst of an attack, it is important to convey some support to the target. If the therapist is working with a cotherapist, the cotherapist must support the target of the coalition. If the therapist is working alone, he must convey the sense that he recognizes the target's side to the story. For example, even as the therapist is helping the husband attack his wife for slovenliness, he interprets the wife's behavior as a resistance to arbitrary control.

When a particular sequence finishes, because a goal has been attained or the threshold of endurance has been reached, the therapist must shift his position and ally with the former target. Sometimes he may even coalesce with him against the former ally.

There is a pitfall to this technique. The family member under attack may counterattack not the therapist, but the family member with whom he is allied. As a result, a family member who is already under severe stress may be overburdened. In the Gorden family, the therapist joins the scapegoated child and defends her by attacking the mother; the mother becomes more aggressive toward her daughter, so the therapist, sensing the increased pressure, moves away from this overly stressful coalition.

The therapist's ultimate goal is to benefit the entire family, and the family must always sense this fact. If he is entering into a coalition against certain family members, they must know that this step is transitional, and that above all, he is allied with the whole family in the therapeutic system.

ASSIGNING TASKS

Tasks create a framework within which the family members must function. The therapist can use tasks to pinpoint and actualize an area of exploration that may not have developed naturally in the flow of family transactions. Or he can highlight an area in which the family needs to work.

Within the Session. Tasks assigned within a session may simply indicate how and to whom family members should communicate. The therapist may say, "Discuss the problem here." He may say, "Talk with your child in such a way that he hears you." Or, "Keep talking; don't let your brother interrupt you."

Tasks can be related to the manipulation of space. The therapist may say, "I want you to turn your chair, so you cannot see your mother's signals." Or, "I want you to sit next to your wife and take her hand whenever you think she is anxious."

Tasks can be used to dramatize family transactions and suggest changes. In one family, the therapist asks the children not to scapegoat one child for three minutes, and he gives his watch to the oldest child to time the interval. In another family, he deputizes the father, saying, "I want you to stop Jim from interrupting Joe during this session." In a family with a hovering mother and a peripheral father, the therapist insists that when he sees the spouses alone, only the father can bring up problems with the children. If the mother wants an issue about the children raised, she has to ask her husband to do it.

By assigning tasks within the session, the therapist highlights his position as the rule setter. It is he who determines the rules of behavior within the therapeutic session.

Homework. The therapist can also assign tasks to be done at home. When the family responds by accomplishing the task he has assigned, they are, in effect, taking the therapist home with them. He becomes the maker of rules beyond the structure of the therapy session.

The task assigned to the Gorden family is aimed both at the presenting problem and the underlying structural problem. The presenting probem is a scapegoated child's fire setting. The therapist instructs the mother to spend five minutes a day with this girl, teaching her how to light matches safely. The parental child, whose helping activities have blocked the scapegoated child from a direct positive contact with her mother, is assigned to watch the other children while the mother works alone with the scapegoated child. In this manner, the therapist ensures that the index patient has some contact each day with a mother who is acting as a competent educator, rather than a scold, and that the parental child is blocked from interfering without losing his position in the family.

In the family with open doors, the task aims at differentiating the family members. In this family, in which the father is allied with the children and the mother is excluded, the therapist asks the wife to determine when the children shall be evicted from the spouses' bedroom and the door closed. The husband is to go along with his wife. The older daughter is to close her door for several hours three times a week. During this time the father must knock at her door if he wants to enter.

In a couple in which the wife controls many aspects of her spouse's life, including his eating manners, his bedtime, and how many times he bathes, the task is aimed at increasing the split between husband and wife, so as to facilitate the restructuring of the spouse subsystem. The husband is asked to buy his clothing by himself for the first time in his life, taking into consideration only his own preferences and tastes. The wife is asked to continue and even to exaggerate her continuous criticism of her spouse, because her husband needs to help her by challenging her irrational authority.

The use of tasks has many advantages. A focus on tasks forces the therapist to deal with the family structure and transactional patterns, rather than with the individual members' particular characteristics. Tasks draw attention to new possibilities for restructuring the family. In formulating tasks, the therapist must clarify his map of the family and establish specific goals as well as specific steps toward these goals. Tasks are also a valuable means of testing family flexibility.

At the same time, the task, like many other therapeutic interventions, is no more than a probe into a family system. The therapist assigning a task does not know how the family members will cope with it. Since he is not committed to the fulfillment of the task, he cannot be disappointed. Giving a task provides a new framework for transactions. The therapist observes the results with a view toward unearthing alternative transactional patterns.

Sometimes a family accepts a task and finds that the alternative behaviors elicited by it are preferable to the old ones—that the family can function better in this expanded range. At other times family members modify the task, contradict it, or avoid it. The different responses give both the therapist and the family a better understanding of where they are and where they must go.

UTILIZING SYMPTOMS

A therapist who is working within the family framework sees an individual member's symptoms as an expression of a contextual problem. Consequently, he may combat the family's tendency to focus on their symptom bearer. In other cases, however, he may choose to work directly with the presenting problems. Sometimes the symptom is so painful or dangerous, such as fire setting, phobia, and anorexia nervosa, that it takes priority. Sometimes the family may be unable at first to make a therapeutic contract that covers anything but the presenting problem.

Focusing on the Symptom. Working with the identified patient's symptoms can often be the quickest route to diagnosing and changing dysfunctional family transactional patterns. The identified patient's symptoms occupy a special position in the family system's lines of transaction. They represent a concentrated nodule of family stress. Frequently, they are one of the family's ways of handling this stress. In any case, the identified patient's symptoms are supported by a number of significant family transactional patterns. Working with them can be, to paraphrase Freud, the royal road to family structure.

In the treatment of the Gorden family, it is obviously urgent to change the presenting problem, fire setting. Also, it is apparent that the fire setting and the transactions around it are a nodule of family stress. Therefore, the therapist does not immediately challenge the family's formulation of the problem. Rather, he follows the strategy of influencing the rest of the family to operate in terms of helping the identified patient in the area of the symptom. While never communicating his own focus on the family structure, he moves the mother from one position in the family structure to another, increasing the mother-daughter proximity while adding distance between that daughter and the parental child, and he does so by using a task based on starting fires.

In the Brown family, the presenting problem, life-threatening anorexia nervosa, is equally urgent, and again it represents a nodule of family stress. The therapist makes the family enact a conflict between parents and child around the symptom, which increases the proximity between the spouses and lessens the protective tie between mother and daughter.

In another case, a child comes into therapy with a dog phobia that is so severe he is almost confined to the house.[2] The therapist's diagnosis is that the symptom is supported by an implicit, unresolved conflict between spouses, manifested in an affiliation between the mother and son that excludes the father. His strategy is to increase the affiliation between the father and son before tackling the spouse subsystem problems. Therefore, he encourages the father, who is a mailman "and therefore an expert in dealing with dogs," to teach his son how to deal with strange dogs. The child, who is adopted, in turn adopts a dog, and the father and son join in transactions around the dog. This activity strengthens their relationship and promotes a separation between mother and son. As the symptom disappears, the therapist praises both parents for their successful handling of the child. He then moves to work with the husband-wife conflicts.

Another therapist encourages a child who soils to maintain his symptom "unless something can happen in the family." He warns the parents to consider carefully what the consequences to themselves would be if the child stopped soiling and "became normal." This procedure, lasting over a month, serves to explore the use of the symptom in the family and reveals the dysfunctional family sets underlying the symptom.

Exaggerating the Symptom. A therapist can use his power within the therapeutic unit to reinforce the identified patient's symptom, increasing its intensity. This tactic becomes a restructuring maneuver.

A middle-aged couple comes into therapy because the husband's depression is so severe that he is unable to work. The therapist, observing the lack of mutual support in this childless couple, interprets the man's depression as a correct assessment of his wasted life and suggests that he mourn for the part of himself that is dead. In accordance with the family's religion, the therapist recommends that the man sit Shiva (the traditional seven days of mourning in Jewish custom) for eight hours a day while his wife brings him food and consoles him. The man cries continually for three days, then becomes bored for four. His depression disappears, and he returns to work. The couple continues treatment in the knowledge that it is not the husband who is depressed, but the entire relationship.

In another family, the presenting problem is the child's stealing. The therapist, who determines that this is a reaction to the lack of effective control in the family, openly instructs the child to continue stealing, and even to steal from his father, saying, "I want to see if you are skillful enough to steal from your father." This device relocates the antisocial behavior in an immediate situation that mobilizes the family's executive controlling functions. The technique is similar to techniques used by A. Aichorn with delinquent children.[3] Again, the deviant behavior of one member becomes an issue of interpersonal regulation in the family.

De-emphasizing the Symptom. At times it is possible to use the symptom as an avenue away from the identified patient. The technique of having lunch with an anorectic patient and his family, for example, facilitates the creation, within the field of eating, of a strong interpersonal conflict, which then takes precedence over the symptom.[4]

In one family composed of a father, mother, and three children aged thirteen, ten, and eight, the father is the identified patient, with psychogenic vomiting. The wife does not want to participate in treatment or allow the children to come. She insists that the problem is the husband's. She does agree, however, to come herself for the initial session. It becomes clear in the session with the couple that the wife is the "owner of rules" in the family. The husband is compliant, except for his vomiting. The thirteen-year-old daughter, from the parents' description of their children, is very anxious, preoccupied with fears that her father will die. The younger son mimics and mocks the father's vomiting. The therapist offers this couple the following choices. He can help the father by teaching him to vomit without making noise, or to limit his vomiting to the bathroom, or even to stop vomiting altogether. But that will not help the couple to acquire mutual respect, or help the two children, on whose lives the parental conflict is encroaching, to learn to individuate. These are the areas it would be more important to treat.

Moving to a New Symptom. The systems concept of the function of a symptom in the family makes it possible to develop a strategy for attacking the identified problem by temporarily moving the focus of therapeutic concentration to another family member. Shifting the focus is used in a family that comes into therapy because of the twelve-year-old son's sleeping disturbance. During therapy, the mother describes her own insomnia of ten years' duration and later indicates her secret pleasure in having company during some of her sleepless nights. Shifting the focus is also used with the Gordens. In the Smith family, the second part of the interview is aimed at moving the skewed label of illness from the husband to the wife.

Relabeling the Symptom. A reconceptualization of the symptom in interpersonal terms can open new pathways for change. In one case, a girl's anorexia is redefined as disobedience and as making her parents incompetent.

Changing the Symptom's Affect. It may be helpful to change the affect of transactions around a symptom. An example is the task given the Gorden girl, which encourages the mother to interact with the child around her problem of fire setting in a competent, educating fashion.

MANIPULATING MOOD

Many families demonstrate a predominant affect. They adhere to a restricted mood level, whatever the content of issues they are discussing. One family will maintain a depressed, apathetic quality; another will constantly tease and joke. The affect accompanying family transactions is one of the many cues that determine the therapist's behavior. Affect is a clue as to what is allowable in a particular family.

Taking on the family's affect is a joining operation, but it can also be a restructuring operation. The therapist can use an exaggerated imitation of the family's style to trigger the family's deviation-countering mechanisms. For example, in a family with an overcontrolling, powerful mother who yells her three adolescent daughters into obedience, the therapist becomes even more aggressive toward them, forcing the mother to soften her mode of contact and to give her daughters more autonomy. In other families, the therapist may wish to demonstrate a different, more appropriate affect. Working with a family concerned with control, for instance, the therapist can adopt a relaxed, accepting mood.[5]

Some families, especially poverty-stricken families or families with a psychosomatically ill member, are so accustomed to emergencies that there is no hierarchy of problems. When a crisis situation arises, its impact is minimized by the feeling of "here we go again." The therapist may have to introduce intensity to make the family respond appropriately to a situation that they should realize is serious. Only by raising the intensity of their response can he trigger their realization that family change is necessary.[6]

Affective components can be used to manipulate distance. In an enmeshed family, a husband accuses his wife of being infantile. Their eleven-year-old boy joins his father, saying, "She is silly when she plays games with me." The therapist indignantly tells the father that he should not tolerate his son's lack of respect for his mother. The therapist's maneuver "lends" indignation to the father, which shames the child. Both the indignation and the shame are distance producing, helping to strengthen the weak boundaries within the family.

Relabeling a predominant affect may also be helpful. If a mother is overcontrolling, the therapist may use the technique of calling her controlling operations "concern" for her children. Such relabeling is frequently only a way of highlighting submerged aspects of the woman's feelings toward her children. The therapist, emphasizing her concern, relates with the mother in a field of sympathy that facilitates the appearance of new transactions between mother and children.

SUPPORT, EDUCATION, AND GUIDANCE

Support, education, and guidance are usually joining operations, but they may also have restructuring functions. The nurturance, healing, and support a family offers its members are vital for the individual family members and for the maintenance of the family system. The therapist must be aware of the importance of these functions and know how to encourage them. Often he may have to teach the family how to confirm each other. He may have to teach parents how to respond differentially to their children. In the family with the open doors, for example, one of the chief aims of the tasks assigned was to provide an experience in differentiated socialization.

If the executive functioning of a family is weak, the therapist may have to enter the system, taking over the executive functions as a model, and then move back so that the parents can reassume these functions. Sometimes the therapist may teach individual family members to deal with the extrafamilial world. For example, a teenaged boy with anorexia nervosa is almost totally isolated from peer group activities. Once the presenting symptom has been cured, the therapist invites the boy to his own home for a week, to visit his teenaged son and daughter. Later, a boy the patient's age who is thoroughly at home in an adolescent peer group is hired to teach the patient how to interact with a group.[7]

A therapist may often teach a child the tricks of getting along in school. When he works with a family in contact with societal agencies that impinge significantly on family life, he may teach them how to handle these agencies as well.

The therapeutic techniques covered here are by no means the only ones a therapist can use. Indeed, large areas have not been been mentioned, such as techniques of working with the family at its interfaces with society. Elie Wiesel wrote that Talmudic tractates traditionally begin with page two, to remind the reader that even if he knows them from one end to the other, he has not even begun.[8] This chapter might well have started on page two, to indicate that even if the reader knows all these techniques thoroughly, he has not even begun.

9 A "Yes, But" Technique: The Smiths and Salvador Minuchin

The Smiths were referred to a family therapist for consultation by a psychiatrist participating in an introductory seminar on family therapy. Mr. Smith has been a psychiatric patient for ten years, having been hospitalized twice for agitated depression. Recently, his symptoms reappeared. He is restless, unable to concentrate, anxious, and has again requested hospitalization. The family interview is an attempt on his psychiatrist's part to find an alternative to hospitalization.

Present at the interview are Mr. Smith, aged forty-nine, his wife, forty-two, their only son Matthew, twelve, and Mrs. Smith's father, Mr. Brown, who has lived with the couple since their marriage. The referring psychiatrist, Dr. Farrell, is also present.

The transcript of the interview itself appears in the left column. In the right column are comments and analysis. The therapeutic strategy and techniques appear in roman type; the thoughts and feelings of the interviewer and the family about both themselves and each other during the session appear in italics. The accommodation and restructuring maneuvers are designated *Ac.* and *Re.*

(*Minuchin is wandering around, re-arranging chairs. He knocks over an ashtray and replaces it.*)

Minuchin: Do you have relatives in Israel?

Ac. Starts the session with a statement that defines him as part of the family's kinship network ("I am like you.")

Mr. Smith: Relatives in Israel? No.

Minuchin: I know a Smith family in Israel. Okay. Let's try to—Dr. Farrell has met only you, and none of the other members of the family.

Ac. Separates himself from the previous therapist. He is a family consultant and may do things differently.

Mrs. Smith: Excuse me, but Dr. Farrell and I had a conversation several years ago. I don't know if you remember. Over at the hospital.

Dr. Farrell: That's right. Only once.

Mrs. Smith: Right.

Dr. Farrell: Mr. Smith was my patient for at least a year or two—

Mr. Smith: I was your patient.

Dr. Farrell: —when I was at the psychiatric clinic. And I left there, oh, I think four or five years ago. Since then, he's been under the care of Dr. Post, who would have liked to be here today but was unable to keep—to make it on such short notice.

Minuchin: You saw Dr. Post weekly?

Mr. Smith: Monthly.

Minuchin. Monthly. What is the problem? You know, I don't know too much about you. And one of the ways in which I work is, I prefer not to know too much, so I didn't ask Dr. Farrell. Probably you will give me your own version of what are the problems, and so we can go out from there. So who wants to start?

Ac. Again, separates himself from the previous therapist, indicating that he will rely on his own hearing of the information the family is now to supply.

Re. Directs his first question about the problem to the whole family, not to the identified patient, which challenges the notion that there is one patient.

Mr. Smith: I think it's my problem. I'm the one that has the problem. And—

Minuchin: Don't be so sure. Never be so sure. (*Mr. Smith is leaning forward, very intent. Minuchin is lounging. Matthew looks at Mr. Smith, and both laugh at Minuchin's reply.*)

Re. Counters Mr. Smith's move to maintain the structure by presenting himself as the problem. The therapist questions the identification of Mr. Smith as the patient and responds to his seriousness with bantering. He also challenges the patient's and family members' reality experience.

Mr. Smith: Well, it seems to be.
Minuchin: Okay.
Mr. Smith: I'm the one that was in the hospital and everything.
Minuchin: Yeah, that doesn't, still, tell me it is your problem. Okay, go ahead. What is your problem?

Re. Challenges the patient's reality again.
Ac. Encourages the identified patient to talk, which keeps him central.

Mr. Smith: Just nervous, upset all the time.
Minuchin: You are upset?
Mr. Smith: Yeah, seem to be never relaxed. Oh, sometimes, sometimes I'm relaxed. But most of the time not. Then I got up tight and I asked them to put me in the hospital. And I have been talking to Dr. Farrell at the hospital.
Minuchin: Do you think that you are the problem?

Ac. and Re. Following the sequence of challenging the husband's claim to his role as a patient, the therapist makes a tracking statement in the form of a question, which carries a restructuring doubt.
Mr. Smith accommodates to the previous attack on the family structure, conceding that someone might be causing his problem.

Mr. Smith: Oh, I kind of think so. I don't know if it's caused by anybody, but I'm the one that has the problem.

Ac. Accommodates to Mr. Smith's accommodation. As a result, a concern for issues of interpersonal causality is now attributed to Mr. Smith The narrow diagnosis is replaced by the broader question: what is the problem?

Minuchin: Mm. If—let's follow your line of thinking. If it would be caused by somebody or something outside of yourself, what would you say your problem is?

Mr. Smith: You know, I'd be very surprised.

Minuchin: Let's think in the family. Who makes you upset?

Mr. Smith counters.

Re: Insists on an interpersonal framework and continues to challenge the identification of Mr. Smith as the problem. At the same time, this approach confirms Mr. Smith's position of centrality in the family. It accommodates to his position as gatekeeper while simultaneously challenging the structure.

Mr. Smith: I don't think anybody in the family makes me upset.

Minuchin: Let me ask your wife. Okay?

Ac. Acknowledges Mr. Smith's position as gatekeeper.

The therapist is experiencing the power of a rigid system, for his challenges have been consistently countered by the identified patient, who insists on remaining the problem. Consequently, the therapist moves to contact another member.

Mr. Smith: Fine. Okay.

Minuchin: Who do you think is—

Mrs. Smith: Well, I've tried to think about it myself, and I really feel he makes his own problems.

Minuchin: Mm.

Mrs. Smith: Because he worries about things like paying the electric bill. That's a normal procedure for every individual. And he has a steady job. He doesn't have to worry about that. He worries about the house. When he comes home—as if the house was going to go away. Well, no one's going to come in and take anything. That's why I say I feel he just makes his own problems. And I really don't feel that I irritate him, unless I don't know about it. Because I always try to go out of my way to do—I try to think like he thinks and will try to do things that—

This long monolog emphasizes the husband's control over his wife and the extent to which she defers to him. But her elaborate description of the ways in which her husband must control her serve to define him as a sick man. As she talks, Mr. Smith displays behavior that underlines the meaning of her communications.

will try to make it easier for him. (*Mr. Smith begins to fidget in rather bizarre ways. He reaches over as if to touch his wife, but lets his hand drop to move along the edge of her chair instead. He "blows off steam" with a long sigh. He examines the corners of his armrest. Suddenly he leans over to extinguish his cigarette, then carefully brushes off every inch of his chair arm. He looks at his watch and examines his fingernails.*) Like for instance, I'll ask him "Well, do you want me to go to the store?" which he says no. He wants to go to the store all the time. "Shall I go down to pay the bills?" No. He wants to. If we get a call to go somewhere, I always say, "Well, I have to ask Bob first." I just don't do it on my own. I always—because I feel he's the head of the family, and this he's entitled to. That I would always ask him before I myself would do anything. So I don't think—

Minuchin: There is nothing that you do that irritates him?

Re. Again questions the validity of labeling the man sick without taking into account the transactional context of the family, and again questions the family member's experience of reality.

Mrs. Smith: Yeah, Well, that's why I say, unless—I don't know. I really don't know. Now, when I first went back to work, about fourteen years ago, is it? Yes, About—approximately fourteen years—

Mr. Smith: Seven—

Mrs. Smith: He didn't like the idea of me going back to work, but when I went back to work, it was because we had a hard time financially, getting along. And he was working two jobs. And at that time he wasn't feeling good, and I said to him, I said, maybe

The therapist's restructuring probes have been deflected by the relentless monolog and by Mr. Smith's symptomatic behavior. The therapist feels curtailed and frustrated; he experiences the need to regain control of the session. However, he cannot interrupt

if I go back to work it would help you. You won't have to work two jobs. And so of course he agreed, but he didn't like me working. But he agreed to it because it was a finance thing at that time. So—

Minuchin: What is your work?

this woman too sharply. That would be construed as another attack on a person already victimized.

Ac. Confirms Mrs. Smith by entering a dialog with her.
Re. As she has been talking about herself only in relation to her husband, the therapist moves her from describing herself as the victim of a sick man to describing her life outside the family.

Mrs. Smith: I work at a bank.
Minuchin: What do you do there?
Mrs. Smith: I'm a file clerk, and I type. Everything in the office, actually. And he—well, he never liked the idea of his wife working. But yet, it made things easier, on the whole. It's not that we're loaded with money, but we don't have to worry about payments.

Again the therapist is blocked. Each spouse has obediently entertained the idea that the husband might not be the sole problem, so they cannot be accused of not cooperating. Mrs. Smith has responded to his attempt to redirect her attention. But after two statements, she returns to describing her husband as a sick man. Within this very rigid system, the therapist's interventions are dropped. The experience of being blocked leads him to develop a new strategy. He realizes that he must join more closely before any restructuring operations can be accepted. He decides to join the spouses by confirming each individually, hoping that he will then be in a position to challenge their interactions. In effect, he will be saying, "You are both nice people, but something in the way you interact is questionable."

Minuchin: Mr. Smith, why don't you like your wife working?

Ac. Makes contact by using the content of Mrs. Smith's monolog.
Re. The terminology "you don't like" is associated with normal behavior, not with being sick.

Mr. Smith: Well, I'm more or less used to it now. But at the time she's talking about, I didn't think a woman should work. And—

Minuchin: Is your family a traditional kind of family?

Mrs. Smith: Oh, yes.

Mr. Smith: Maybe it's because Mother never worked. I mean, outside of the house, she never worked. And I always wanted to do the supporting, and—

Minuchin: That your wife worked meant something? That you could not support her?

Mr. Smith: At the time that she said, I was working two jobs. And I was complaining a little bit. And that's why she said she would do—

Minuchin: What's your work?

Re. Interrupts a train of thought headed toward again making the point that Mr. Smith is sick, turning it into a dialog about other areas.

Mr. Smith: Where do I work? I work for a manufacturer.

Minuchin: What is your job? What do you do?

Mr. Smith: I work in the lab as a technician and an inspector.

Minuchin: That means the production aspect of it?

Ac. Although the therapist does not understand and is not interested in Mr. Smith's work, his question opens up a common area; they can talk about business together.

Re. The content is about normal aspects of the identified patient's life.

Mr. Smith: Well, on overtime I work in production. During the week I work right in the lab, working on samples and different tests to be made. We use the microscope a lot, reading samples under a microscope.

Minuchin: How long have you been working there?

Ac. Exploring the man's life confirms him.

Re. Continues to emphasize the normal aspects of life.

Mr. Smith: Thirty years.
Minuchin: Thirty years! My goodness!
Mr. Smith: Yeah. With the company. But not in this job thirty years. Just about seven years on this job.
Minuchin: I don't know. I never worked any place more than seven years. This is the longest time I have worked. I am much more restless than you, clearly. I am a very restless kind of person. (*He scratches his head, checks his watch, and fiddles with his coat.*)

Ac. Becomes less assertive, mimicking Mr. Smith, and introduces his own personal life, talking as worker to worker.

Re. By joining Mr. Smith, the therapist suggests that the patient may not be sick. Furthermore, by becoming "restless," the therapist creates a paradoxical situation in which the weaker man, Mr. Smith, is seen as the stronger. If such confusion is possible, the identified patient's sickness may also be open to question. The rigidity of the family's schema is questioned.
The therapist is aware of pursuing a strategy that will enable him to get closer to Mr. Smith. He is not aware that his behavior is fumbling and that his stance has lost power. He uses talking about himself as a means both of getting closer and of challenging the definition of the man as sick. He feels more accepted, more relaxed, and more confident that his interventions will now be accepted by the system.

Mr. Smith: Mm.
Minuchin: You are not, evidently.

Re. Insists on making his message explicit.

Mr. Smith: No, I wouldn't say I'm restless. I mean, I sleep. But I don't—
Minuchin: But you are steady in one—
Mr. Smith: As far as the job's concerned, yeah. Well, I went there at nineteen, and I've stayed down there.

Ac. Confirms Mr. Smith as competent.

Minuchin: You are now forty-nine?
Mr. Smith: Forty-nine.
Minuchin (hesitates, as if thinking): We are the same age.

Mr. Smith: Are we?

Minuchin: And when did you begin to kind of worry about things?

Mr. Smith: Ten years ago.
Minuchin: Ten years. Tell me, maybe your son—your only son?
Mr. Smith: Yeah.
Minuchin (to Matthew): Your father said he is the problem, and your mother agrees that he is the problem in the family. But what are the things that make your father—that irritate him, that make him upset, so he gets pissed off?

Ac. The therapist and Mr. Smith are similar in age as well as in restlessness and in being workers.
Mr. Smith acknowledges, accommodating to the therapist.
Re. Now disengages, becoming the expert addressing a person in need of help.

Ac. Establishes that he has Mr. Smith's permission to contact Matthew.

Ac. Keeps the father in the position of identified patient as he contacts his son.
Re. To explore the interpersonal transactions that may irritate Mr. Smith questions the presenting problem of intrapsychic pathology.
Having successfully established contact with two family members, the therapist moves to include a third. He uses language geared to an adolescent, approaching him as a person who observes things in the family.

Matthew: I don't know. I don't think it's like—anybody that puts it on him. It's just—I don't know.

When Minuchin contacted Matthew, he hoped to find an ally—a pathway for restructuring interventions. Instead, the boy parrots his mother. The therapist is irritated, and his frustration becomes part of his next communication to the family.
Re. Insists that the family explore interpersonal transactions. The therapist challenged the system only indirectly while talking with the father and mother, but while talking with the son, he attacks strongly. Again he questions a family member's perception of reality.

Minuchin: I just can't believe that, you know. People are always part of—when people live together, then they irritate each other, you know. I am sure your father irritates you sometimes. *(Mrs. Smith nods emphatically.)* And I am sure that your grandfather irritates you sometimes. And you in turn irritate your grandfather and your mother and father. I am sure of that. Am I right?

Ac. Finishes his attack with a request for affiliation and acknowledgment.

Matthew: Yeah. But I don't irritate him that much, like really nervous. I might, you know, be bad sometimes. But I don't think I really irritate him that much.

Minuchin: What about your grandpa? Does he irritate your father?

Ac. Addresses boy as a competent observer of the family scene.

Matthew: No. He don't say much.

Minuchin: Grandpa doesn't say much. How old are you, Mr. Brown?

Ac. Makes contact with the fourth member, affiliating with him jovially.

Mr. Brown: I don't know. Sometimes I think I say too much.

Minuchin: How old are you?

Mr. Brown: How much do you think?

Minuchin: Oh, like fifty-three.

Mr. Brown: Seventy-eight.

Minuchin: Seventy-eight. You look fine.

The therapist feels a sense of respect for the elderly. He also feels protective toward the grandfather, sensing his displacement in the family.
The grandfather also maintains the family structure.

Mr. Brown: No, I'll tell you now what I think. What brings it on is Bob himself. He's always worried about me. He wants everything done just certain ways, see? He's particular, in other words, see? And he sees something ain't done, and right away, he's got to go and do it. And someone says, "I'll do it." "No, I'll do it. I'll do it," he says. That's one thing, now. Now, another—

Minuchin: You are saying he likes to do things instead—for other people?

Re. Relabels Mr. Brown's description of Mr. Smith's actions. Mr. Brown calls them controlling; the therapist suggests they are helpful.
Mr. Smith insists on his position as a patient. He interrupts the dialog between Mr. Brown and Minuchin, eliciting a structure-maintaining communication from the grandfather.

Mr. Smith: I think he missed the point.

Mr. Brown: No, no, no. For himself. Now, suppose there's dirt on the carpet or something like that. He'd say, "Well, there's dirt on the carpet." She'd say, "I'll clean it up." "Never mind, I'll do it." And he'd go right away and clean it up. Now I don't think he should do that.

Minuchin: He's helpful that way.

Mr. Brown: I don't think it's good. I don't think he should do that. There's lots of things that he does that he shouldn't do. He should let someone else do something too.

Minuchin: Like who?

Mr. Brown: Any one of the three of us.

Minuchin: He takes everything on his shoulders?

Mr. Brown: Almost everything. I— pretty near everything.

Minuchin: You—what's your name, you said?

Matthew: Matthew.

Minuchin: Matthew. You disagreed with that—with your grandfather's statement.

Matthew: I think he's partly right. I don't think he takes that—you know. He does try to do a lot of things. Like, somebody will offer. He'll say, "No, I can do it myself." I don't feel like he takes everything on. He'll do a lot of that. Not really too much. But he tells me to take out the trash and all, still. Stuff like that, I still got to do most of.

Mrs. Smith: But then when you don't do it, he ends up doing it.

Re. Again relabels.

Mr. Brown seems genuinely concerned for Mr. Smith, not just in alliance with his daughter. But the grandfather is not powerful in the system. The therapist treats him with respect but decides that restructuring interventions utilizing the grandfather cannot succeed.

Ac.

Ac. Having established affiliation with Mr. Brown, turns back to another member and seeks contact with Matthew in a more familiar mode.

Matthew's complaint sounds quite typical of problems between adolescent sons and their fathers. Mrs. Smith joins in an alliance with Mr. Smith, defining the boundaries of the parental subsystem.

Mr. Smith: I don't think that's what's wrong, because I don't—I could help my wife more as far as cleaning is concerned.

Matthew: Yeah, like he'll come home and, like, run the carpet sweeper.

Mr. Smith: Just fast stuff.

Matthew: Yeah.

Mrs. Smith: But it's a big help.

Mr. Smith: Heavy cleaning, I don't do for her, and dishes, I don't do for her. Yeah, I do help her with the dishes ever since I've been married, but not all the time. Most of the time.

Matthew: I think he means like if something's, like, broken in the house, or—

Minuchin (indignantly): Wait a moment, wait a moment. Who means?

Matthew: My grandfather.

Minuchin: Your grandfather. You are explaining your grandfather.

Matthew: Yeah. Like if something's broken in the house or something, he'll want to do it himself, or something.

Mr. Smith: No, I'm not too handy a person that way. I want it done right away, probably, and characteristic—

Matthew: Yeah, like you want it done right away.

Mrs. Smith: He hasn't enough patience to wait.

Mrs. Smith: But I don't think that's bad. A lot of people are that way.

Mr. Smith re-establishes his position as sick and reactivates his son's treatment of him as sick.

Re. Models for Mr. Smith a way of defining the intergenerational boundary, for indignation is a powerful force for separation.

The therapist feels that Matthew criticizes his father too freely, so he decides to attack the son, showing his indignation.

All three statements maintain Mr. Smith as sick. There is agreement on this dysfunctional transactional pattern, which keeps the family close. Mr. Smith had again started to portray himself as sick, which activates Mrs. Smith's protectiveness, preventing further amplification.

Minuchin: Mom was saying, "Don't be critical of Dad."

Ac. Maintains and defines the spouse subsystem boundary so that support-ive, positive transactions can grow. *The therapist feels he has been too negative toward Mrs. Smith and cor-rects himself.*

Matthew: She what?

Minuchin: She just said, "Don't be critical of Daddy." Because you were saying, "He's impatient," and Mom says, "Well, you know, a lot of people are like that." Is she protective of Father?

Ac.

Matthew: I don't think so.

Minuchin: There is nothing wrong with that. I think it is rather nice.

Ac. Again supports spouse subsystem, dwelling on positive husband-wife trans-actions, which reassures Matthew that he does not have to be involved.

Matthew: She is a little bit, I guess. I don't think she's really overprotec-tive.

Minuchin: I just mean protective, in a nice way. In the same way in which Daddy apparently is protective of everybody else, according to Grandpa. Is that true? Is your husband trying to do things, trying to do your job?

Ac. Confirms Mr. and Mrs. Smith as positive and good.
Re. Emphasizing positives in the husband-wife relationship challenges the family schema.

Mrs. Smith: Well, he worries about me excessively.

(Mr. Smith sighs loudly, then suddenly springs up, strips off his jacket, and strides away to hang it up. Then he lights a cigarette.)

The therapist feels that he is losing Mr. Smith, who has a glassy, distant look in his eyes. He feels a need to be in contact with Mr. Smith, but Mrs. Smith continues talking and he does not want to interrupt her rudely.

Minuchin: He worries about you. That you don't like?

Mrs. Smith: Yes. I don't think he should, because I feel I'm an individual, and he shouldn't worry so much. Be-cause he has a lot of his own problems he should take care of.

Mrs. Smith's remark about Mr. Smith's problems is a distancing communica-tion, made in response to the thera-pist's previous operation, which was designed to increase husband-wife contact.

Minuchin: You mean he worries about you, sometimes it bothers you. Can I have a cigarette, Mr. Smith?

Mr. Smith: Sure (*offers a cigarette to the therapist*).

Minuchin: I smoke only when I just don't know what to do, but by this time I don't know what to do, so I am worried. I am smoking. (*The therapist takes off his coat, hangs it up, and walks back to get a light from Mr. Smith.*)

Re. Counters Mrs. Smith's attempt to maintain the prevailing structure with an interpersonal confirmation supporting the husband-wife subsystem.

Ac.
These are spontaneous mimetic operations, resulting from the therapist's concern. Mr. Smith's symptomatic behavior and Mrs. Smith's distancing operation have again left the therapist feeling excluded and powerless. The therapist and Mr. Smith are now both smoking and both in their shirtsleeves.

Ac. Tries to decrease distance by using first names.

Minuchin: What's your wife's name?

Mr. Smith: Rosemary.

Minuchin: Rosemary. And yours?

Mr. Smith: Bob. Robert.

Minuchin: Bob. Rosemary says that sometimes you worry too much about her. What does she mean?

The therapist has retraced his steps, having observed that direct contact with Mrs. Smith activates Mr. Smith's restlessness. He now contacts the wife through the husband. Having accommodated by honoring Mr. Smith's centrality, and mimicked by taking off his coat and lighting a cigarette, Minuchin once more feels in contact with Mr. Smith.

Mr. Smith: Well, I'm—I don't really know what she means by that. I'm concerned over her, and I'm very much in love with her, and I don't think I worry too much.

Minuchin: Let's find out. Let's find out. (*He gestures, indicating that Mr. Smith and Mrs. Smith should talk.*)

Re. Assigns task of talking to each other.

The therapist senses that the family members will now follow his instructions, so he starts a different phase of the interview, instructing the partici-

pants to talk to each other so as to activate their enactment of accustomed transactional patterns. He now wants to keep himself out of the discussion as much as possible.

Mr. Smith: I don't know what you mean by—

Mrs. Smith (speaking mostly without looking at Mr. Smith): Well, sometimes actually, like when I come home from work or something, for instance Saturday. Well, maybe not Saturday. Any day.

Mr. Smith: M-hm.

Minuchin: You know something? You have that chair, that one, in the middle, kind of between you. (*He moves the chair out.*)

Re. Continues challenging the distancing mechanisms of husband and wife by using space redistribution.

Mr. Smith: Started being more, uh— (*He shifts his chair.*)

Minuchin: Yeah.

Mrs. Smith: He questions, like, all my movements, and it's nothing that—

Minuchin: Can you look at—can you turn your chair?

Re. Increases the intensity of his probe.

Mr. Smith: Turn my chair?

Minuchin: Yeah. Just so that you can look at her. (*He gets up and helps spouses change the angle of their chairs so they are facing each other.*)

Re. Continues to change spatial arrangements, increasing the stress in the husband-wife subsystem, which may encourage the unfolding of alternative transactional patterns.

Mr. Smith: Yeah.

Minuchin: Because maybe you don't —you miss some of the messages.

Ac. Acknowledges Mr. Smith as he explains the reason for the request. The increase in stress is thus accompanied by a supportive statement.

Mr. Smith: The last twenty-three years.

Mrs. Smith (laughs): No, but like, he'll always—it's very hard to explain. I really don't know how to explain it.

Mr. Smith: I think that she means—

Both spouses are maintaining the preferred transactional pattern, talking to the therapist instead of to each other.

Minuchin: No, no. no. (*He gestures indicating they should talk to each other.*)

Mrs. Smith: No, but he's always—

Minuchin: Tell him. Tell him. Tell him.

Mrs. Smith: All right. Like when I come home, "What did this one say, what did that one say?" That's when I go to the hairdresser's. When you go somewhere and see somebody and see Mary, or somebody, and I'll say "What did Mary say"—which is nothing wrong when you ask me. But yet, at the same time, he don't tell me. But yet in another respect, like if I'm sick, he'll come home from work and I'll be laying up in bed, and I'll be waiting, waiting for you to come up to see how I am. And you don't come up. You'll sit down and have a beer and a cigarette, and then decide to come up. And I—remember when I was in the hospital? What a hard time you gave me in the hospital? You—you vary. I just don't know how to explain it, really.

Mr. Smith: Yeah.

Mrs. Smith: And yet, I know he—you love me, and I love you. But—maybe that's the problem. Maybe you don't know how to show love. You think that could be it?

Mr. Smith (to Minuchin): All right to answer?

Minuchin: Yeah. Yeah, please. Answer to her. She asked you a question.

Mr. Smith: M-hm. I don't think that's good reasoning there. I don't think that's not a problem. But I don't think that's my problem. I know I get concerned a lot of times about your personal things, which I don't think you like, and which I shouldn't be concerned about. But, well, I mean, she—

Re. Insists that they talk to each other, excluding the therapist.

Another pattern has appeared in response to the decreased distance between the spouses and the firming of the boundary around the spouse subsystem. It is not the concern of a wife for her sick husband, but the complaint of a wife about a selfish, controlling man.

Re. Reinforces spouse subsystem boundary.

Mr. Smith is trying to re-establish the preferred transactional pattern, with himself as the sick member. He addresses himself to the therapist, drawing him into the spouse conflict as a way of increasing the distance. He also placates his wife from his usual position of weakness.

it is true. I've come home and I knew she was sick and I didn't go right up but—

Minuchin: Bob. Rosemary asked you a question. You don't need to answer me, because she asked you a question. So you answer.

Mr. Smith: What was your question?

Mrs. Smith: Oh, I forgot it now because I think there were so many other things.

Dr. Farrell: You said maybe he doesn't know how to show love.

Mrs. Smith: Oh. That's right. Maybe that's what it is.

Dr. Farrell: Yes.

Mrs. Smith: You think that's the problem? That even though, like I know you love me, because every once in a while you do tell me (*Minuchin laughs*). But yet you don't know how to show it.

Minuchin: That's funny.

Mrs. Smith: Really. And yet to me these are the little things that mean a lot to me.

Minuchin: Of course.

Mr. Smith: It's a good question. How do you show love? How can you show it? In material things, or in—

Mrs. Smith: Well, I don't think you show it in material things. I don't believe you show it in material things. I think you show love by doing for one another and go out of your way to help one another, making it easy for one another. This is my opinion. And maybe you have a different opinion about it.

Re. Reinforces boundary.

The therapist thinks this statement is very funny, starts to laugh, and suddenly finds his laughter inappropriate because it does not communicate to any of the family members.

Mr. Smith: Well, I think we're getting off the problem.

Mr. Smith feels uncomfortable with the decreased distance and the appearance of interpersonal problems between him and his wife.

Mrs. Smith: No, we were talking about—

Minuchin: Maybe we are getting near the problem instead of off the problem. I am interested in knowing how you two people get along together.

Re. Reinforces boundaries and keeps the problem at the interpersonal level.

Mrs. Smith: Well, Bob doesn't have too much to say, In fact, I'm always telling him, "How come you're so quiet?"

Activated by her husband's previous statement, the wife again addresses herself to the therapist, lessening the strength of the spouse subsystem boundary.

Mr. Smith: I don't have too much—

Mrs. Smith: He doesn't talk much. I do most of the talking, and half the time I don't think he even hears me. Yet if I say, "Did you hear what I said?" "Yeah, I heard what you said." Right?

The wife interrupts her husband when he starts to talk, maintaining him in the position of the silent member while she is complaining of his silence.

Dr. Farrell: You said something about him giving you a hard time in the hospital?

Mrs. Smith: M-hm.

Mr. Smith: Not the last time you was in.

Mrs. Smith: Well, not the last time, because we had it straightened out. But I have a herniated disc, and the doctor wanted me to stay for eighteen days. No. I forget how long. Excuse me, I forgot how long.

Mr. Smith: You had been in about two weeks.

She uses her husband for a memory bank, reinforcing his control over her.

Mrs. Smith: Yeah, I had been in. But even when I went in the first week, he got very upset because I went in. And he called the doctor and wanted me to come out, and would call me on the phone and really insist that I come out, because he thought I could lay at home in traction just as well as I could lay in the hospital in traction. And my doctor even talked to Bob, and he said he couldn't make Bob understand it. He said it was like talking to a wall. He just wanted me to be home with him. So then finally it had to be that I had to go home, and I really asked the doctor if he would please let me go home and rig up the traction and stuff at the house, and then Bob was satisfied, then.

(*Minuchin shifts position, brushes off the table, and fidgets.*)

The wife, talking to the therapist about her husband, has spread her complaints. The effect is to shift back to a focus on his sickness. The therapist is showing impatience with the length of her speech.

Mr. Smith: I think that was a case of where I thought what she said could be done at home. She was just laying in traction at the hospital, and—and I guess I should have kept quiet. It's one time I was talking. But that's been three or four years.

Mrs. Smith: Three years ago.

Minuchin: You moved from center. He was saying—you were asking some questions to Bob, and you were trying to answer. You know, I always think, Bob, that if you are having some difficulties, I always try to find out what the heck is going on between you and your wife. So these are the kind of things I would like us to look at now. Okay?

Re. Reassigns the task of exploring interpersonal issues within the dyad. The therapist, having experienced this family system's great resistance to change, begins to intervene more insistently, in order to further the task. *The therapist thinks that Mr. Smith deflects all of his wife's criticisms by apologizing and stating his incompetence. He decides to probe by encouraging Mr. Smith to stand up to his wife, promoting conflict.*

Mrs. Smith: M-hm.

Minuchin: Because it seems to me that Rosemary is—was expressing some critical opinions just now, you know. And maybe she wants you to answer some of these things.

Ac. Supports the wife's complaints while talking to the husband in a friendly way.

Mrs. Smith: Well, I have already asked him these things before.

Minuchin: Ask him now.

Mrs. Smith: Like I—remember, you always have to go in and look at my clothes, checking my clothes to see if everything's there, open my drawers, which I don't think—it's not that I don't think that you shouldn't. Well, I don't feel that you should do it. And yet I'm not mad because you do it.

Minuchin: Oh, you are, Rosemary. You are mad. Don't tell me you aren't mad.

Mrs. Smith: No, well, let me explain it further, please. Because I feel that these are my things, and I don't go— because he has told me. He won't even let me dust his bureau because I can't move anything out of place. But he's always going in my drawers, making sure that everything's there, as if I'm going to give it away to someone. I'm not going to give anything away. And I've asked him many times, why do you have to check on my clothes and my possessions?

(Minuchin walks behind Mr. Smith and makes him shift his chair so that he faces his wife even more directly. Minuchin sits next to the man. Mr. Smith moves the wastebasket so it is between him and Minuchin and stubs out a cigarette in the wastebasket. Minuchin moves back a little.)

Mr. Smith: I think it's just a habit.

Mrs. Smith: But yet you don't want me to do yours, and you won't even let me dust the bureau. Why?

Mr. Smith: I don't know why. I think it's because I have things memorized like in—which is—I don't know if it's normal or not. And you're

Mrs. Smith refuses the task, talking with the therapist.

Re. Promotes conflict.

Re. Curtails the preferred transactional pattern that maintains Mr. Smith as the patient and isolates husband and wife. By maintaining the stress of husband-wife proximity, the therapist facilitates the appearance of conflict, which frees Mr. Smith from the deviant position. Now he looks like a garden-variety selfish husband.

right. I have gotten mad when she's moved my papers and stuff. And I just thought that I can dust the bureau myself, that's all.

Mrs. Smith: Yeah, but it hasn't been dusted in a long time. And this is what makes me mad, then, because when he looks at—when you look at my things. Because you don't let me look at your things.

Mrs. Smith has accommodated to the therapist's demand for increased strength in the spouse subsystem boundary. At the point where she would ordinarily bring in another person, she begins to bring in the therapist. Then, instead of using the therapist to deflect spouse conflict, she continues to confront her husband.

Mr. Smith: I don't care if you've been in the drawer or not. (*He is avoiding his wife's eyes. Minuchin taps his shoulder and indicates that he should look at her.*)

Mrs. Smith: If it hadn't been for that, then I don't think I would have been mad. But under these circumstances, is why I get mad. You should—if one can do it, why can't the other do it?

Mr. Smith: If you want to go in my drawers, I don't care.

Mrs. Smith: That's how I feel. But yet you get so burned up, you know.

Mr. Smith: I don't really get burned up.

Mrs. Smith: Oh, Bob. You really yell. You know you do. Be honest.

Mr. Smith: I don't think I get mad—

Mr. Smith is trying to maintain the system by placating his wife. She does not respond to his indications that they have reached the limit of allowed disagreement and it is time to deflect; she continues to confront him. The husband retreats.

Minuchin: Does she have a big temper?

Ac. Joins Mr. Smith by criticizing his wife. Supporting the husband in a coalition against his wife will also continue the conflict.

Mr. Smith: No, we've had—

Minuchin: No, she. She.

Re. Allows no retreat.

Mr. Smith: No, she doesn't.

Mrs. Smith: Oh, I scream now. I scream.

Mr. Smith: Aw, for a minute you'll scream.

Minuchin: You are hiding that she has a big temper.

Mr. Smith: No, I never thought she had a big temper.

Minuchin: Oh, I see it here, you know. She is like pepper. Like pepper, she is quite able to get—

Mr. Smith: She can express herself all right.

Minuchin: She gets quite excited, doesn't she?

The therapist has realized that his attack must be more direct, since Mr. Smith will not by himself attack his wife. The therapist is also reacting to the quick deflection of his probes, even after he had begun to think they were leading somewhere.

Mr. Smith: I don't think so. You think so?

Mrs. Smith: I think so.

Minuchin: Oh, yeah.

Mr. Smith: Are we on television?

Confronted by an alliance of his wife and the therapist, which is working toward a spouse subsystem confrontation, Mr. Smith jumps outside the context and becomes preoccupied with the TV cameras, which were explained to him before the session. This is an indication that the threshold of pressure which Mr. Smith can tolerate is being reached.

As the session continues, the therapist's immediate goal, sparked by Mr. Smith's panic, is to accommodate further to Mr. Smith before continuing his explorations. Conflictual material unfolds. Mr. Smith reveals that at some time he felt the grandfather was occupying too much space in their life, but he did not make this clear. Mr. Smith considers himself a very angry man, able to do damage if he lets his temper go. Mrs. Smith agrees, saying his temper frightens her.

The pattern of the conflicts so far unfolded repeats itself. Mrs. Smith complains, Mr. Smith denies, Mrs. Smith interrupts him, and he placates her by indicating his inadequacy. Or Mrs. Smith complains, and Mr. Smith agrees with her that he should have acted differently. Whenever the therapist challenges Mr. Smith's view of himself as sick and his wife as well, or criticizes Mrs. Smith, Mr. Smith responds with some indication of his inadequacy. Again and again, the therapist's inputs are disqualified by Mr. Smith, though not by Mrs. Smith.

The next segment occurs about half an hour later. Minuchin has asked Mr. Brown and Matthew to leave the room and turned the conversation to the couple's sex life, about which they are evasive.

Minuchin: Is there any way you are critical of Rosemary?

Re. Tries to elicit criticism from Mr. Smith that would balance the skewed husband-wife arrangement.

Mr. Smith: Critical of her? Do you think I'm critical of you?
Mrs. Smith: I don't know, Bob; he asked you. I don't know.

Mrs. Smith has accommodated more to the therapist, but the system, with its rigid transactional patterns, maintains itself.

Mr. Smith: If she wants to go somewhere, I—
Minuchin: I am asking if there is anything—I know that she is critical of you. I am asking, are you critical of anything about Rosemary. Do you want her to change in any way?
Mr. Smith: No.
Minuchin: Hm?
Mr. Smith: No, I don't believe so. I love her the way she is. And—
Minuchin: Dr. Farrell has sent me a little note here. It says that Mrs. Smith has never been sexually responsive. And I don't know—

The therapist, having felt himself disqualified time after time, has now developed a strategy for intervening in the skewed husband-wife relationship. He will put all his weight behind seeing the wife as sick. This can be done only by a close coalition between him and

*the reluctant Mr. Smith. Transitional
transactional patterns based on this
strategy will increase the utilization of
alternative patterns in this rigid system.*

Mr. Smith: Well, I thought we were
going to get to that. I have talked to
Dr. Farrell. We have touched on this
subject. She's just—and I've talked with
my wife. She's just what I'd call a cold-
natured person. Oh, she's not very—I
don't know what the word is—sexually
inclined, which years ago, I used to be
very concerned about. But I've more or
less taken to accept it now. And—
maybe because I've gotten older and
my sexual drive is lessened too. But we
at times had a sex problem, and I used
to ask her to go to the doctor about it,
and she did mention it to our family
doctor and—this was a few years back.
And—but I've more or less gotten to
accept it. I mean, I didn't think it was
grounds for a divorce or nothing. Other
things—I thought there was other
things in the world besides sex too.
Because that's a very big part of
married life—

Minuchin: But you did have sex.

Mr. Smith: Yeah. Well, I mean, you
people are doctors. She's never denied
me the right. It's just that she doesn't
get into it very much. And the last few
years, I began to believe that it's on
account of the way I've been feeling
and everything. You have to be in a
good mood, to have sex and everything.
And—it's a pretty difficult subject to
talk on.

Minuchin: When was the last time
you two had sex?   *Ac.* Supports Mr. Smith.

Mr. Smith: The last time? Uh, I guess
it was right before I come in the
hospital. But I don't know if there's a

normal set rule on having sex or if
there's just whenever you feel the
urge.

Minuchin: Hm. How frequently do
you feel the urge?

Mr. Smith: Well, years ago I—I used
to feel the urge every night. But in the
last year or two maybe once every two
weeks or something. I have these other
things in my mind. I think if it wasn't
for that, I probably would be thinking
about that maybe more often.

*Mr. Smith has begun to accommodate
to the therapist. He is close to making
a connection between his present
symptoms and his interpersonal problems with his wife.*

Minuchin: And what happened to
Rosemary? What happened to you?
You just don't care?

Re. To emphasize Mr. Smith's normality and potentials while exploring
Mrs. Smith as the problem, the therapist's question is slightly derogatory.

Mrs. Smith: I just—I never—I don't
know. The doctor told me when I went
to him—like we have this problem—
and he said that I'm a highly nervous
person and that I have to be relaxed. I
don't know how to relax. And that was
the problem. In fact, at that particular
time, if you remember, Bob, he suggested that I take a cocktail or something in the evening to sort of relax me.
Which has seemed to help. But everything has to go smooth. Like, before
we go to bed, I can't have any upsets.
If I get all upset, then I can't seem to
get in the mood.

Minuchin: What happens when you
are not in the mood and he is in the
mood? What happens?

Ac. Tracking.
Re. Explores conflict, with the wife
now as the deviant.

Mrs. Smith: Well, I always let him
come. Always let him hold me, and—
you know. Even though I don't come.

Minuchin: And he feels like you
don't care for him when that happens.

Re. Manipulates affect, "lending"
feelings of rejection and anger to Mr.
Smith.
*The therapist, working in coalition
with Mr. Smith, feels annoyed with
him for not protecting himself. His
anger is actualized as an attack on Mrs.
Smith.*

Mrs. Smith: I don't get that feeling.
Minuchin: Okay.
Dr. Farrell: He told me he used to get very mad about it, when you-all were younger. You weren't aware of it?
Mrs. Smith: Because he would get in the mood every night, like he said, and I just couldn't get in the mood because if I were tired, or something, that day—like I said, I'm the type of a person that everything has to go real smooth. And I can't have any upsets because when I get upset, I can't—and that's why I went to the doctor.
Mr. Smith: Well, maybe at one time that was my biggest problem, which I knew it was normal to have a problem like that.
Minuchin: You are a person with a strong sexual urge.

Ac. Emphasizes Mr. Smith's power.

Mr. Smith: Well, I agree with you now. Maybe that had something to do with bringing on the condition I had, if I want to throw it off on somebody else. Because I know at the time I used to just look forward to coming home and having sex with my wife, you know, before she went to work. And it used to irritate me a lot.

Mr. Smith agrees with the therapist's view of complementarity between his problem and his wife's.

Minuchin: You like to hold her, and you like to kiss?
Mr. Smith: Yeah. Yeah.
Mrs. Smith: I'd like to get it straightened out.

Mrs. Smith accepts the label of sick.

Minuchin: Apparently there is a part of Bob, the romantic part of Bob, that feels you don't accept part of him.

Re. In the middle of the session, the therapist tried to have Mr. Smith confront his wife. Now he confronts her himself, acting as Mr. Smith's proxy. Mrs. Smith accepts the therapist as the voice of her husband.

Later in the session, Mrs. Smith again describes her husband. Confronted by the powerful coalition of her husband and the therapist, she responds with an attack on her husband, the weaker member of the coalition. The familiar transactional pattern begins. Mr. Smith placates, while Mrs. Smith ignores him and continues complaining. But there is a small sign of change, for caught between having to placate his wife and having to accommodate to his ally, the therapist, Mr. Smith suggests a disqualification of his helpless stance. The pattern emerges as follows.

Mrs. Smith: But he doesn't—see, this is what I feel is wrong. It is our house in black and white. But I don't feel that it is my house. I'm afraid to invite people up because I feel Bob—it's just like he said a few minutes ago about when he gets mad, he really gets mad. And I'm always afraid of upsetting him. And like, a lot of my friends, he don't like, I don't invite them. Because I know he gets mad. So I don't even invite them.	*Attack.*
Minuchin: I don't think you are so afraid of him.	
Mrs. Smith: Oh, I am. When he gets mad, I—I'm scared of him.	
Mr. Smith: When—who's your friends I don't like?	*Defense.*
Mrs. Smith: Well, you don't like when Martha comes up. You put—you say you put up with them. But you don't talk to them. You never like Ann. You never seem to care for her.	*Attack.*
Mr. Smith: Well, I always liked Joanne.	*Defense.*
Mrs. Smith: And when Barbara used to come—but yet when your friends, especially the fellows from where you work—when they come, you bend over backwards. And when they come to our house, I'm always nice to them. I always try and go out of my way.	*Continued attack, without acknowledging the defense.*
Mr. Smith: Hold on, hold on a—	*Attempt to defend.*

Mrs. Smith: But yet you don't do that for my friends.

Continued attack without acknowledgment, but shifting the focus.

Mr. Smith: I'm not a good conversationalist, I know that.

Defense of incompetence.

Mrs. Smith: Yeah, but you are with your friends, Bob.

Acknowledgment and support.

Mr. Smith: Well, I don't have as much in common with your friends as the people I work with. But I—
the doctor disagrees with me—
—I don't think that's the root of my problem. It may indirectly be.
But what gives me the urge to do the things I do? It's like an urge.

Defense in interpersonal terms.

Accommodation to therapist.
System maintenance.
Accommodation to therapist.
System maintenance.

At the end of the hour, Minuchin summarizes for the couple, indicating that their problem is interpersonal, and the therapeutic unit will continue working from that premise.)

Mr. Smith: You think my problem lays there?

Minuchin: I don't know. But I would think your problem lies here, between you two. You put it all inside of you. But it is here. And you are not looking at that. You are not looking at the way in which you two treat each other. You see, you have accepted—both of you have accepted—that it's easier if you say, "It's my fault," than if you look at what's happening to both of you. Why is it easier to say, "It's my fault," instead of saying, "Rosemary, it's something of the way in which we are dancing together. Just, there is no music to it." You know, that's what you are saying. There is no music to that dance. We will stop here. But you see, Dr. Farrell, I am convinced that you cannot help Bob at all unless Rosemary changes. You know. And that he will not be helpful. Because he prefers to say, "It's my fault," than to talk with his wife.

Dr. Farrell: M-hm.

Mrs. Smith: I don't know how to change.

Minuchin: No, it's you, Bob, that needs to change her.

Mr. Smith: I never thought it was her fault.

Minuchin: Of course. It's easier if you think it's your fault. Will you do it to her, or not?

Mr. Smith: What? Try to change her?

Minuchin: Yeah.

Mr. Smith: It takes a lot of thought.

Minuchin: No, it doesn't take thought. It takes—it needs doing, man. Okay?

Mr. Smith: Right.

Mrs. Smith accepts her role as sick.

Re. Indicates a task: Mr. Smith is to change Mrs. Smith.

In this family, there is an agreement that Mr. Smith is the problem. He is the most vocal supporter of his position in the family. The very rigid family structure has been reinforced by the ten years of medical concurrence that Mr. Smith is mentally ill.

Minuchin's strategems are related to the goal of freeing Mr. Smith from the deviant position. In order to do this, he first attenuates Mr. Smith's experience that he is the deviant. He then challenges the validity of that experience in both Mr. Smith and his family.

His first challenge is based on the metaphor of Alice's room. If Alice's room grows while Alice stays the same, Alice will experience change. Therefore, Minuchin imitates Mr. Smith. The movements made by Mr. Smith to reaffirm that he is the deviant are mimicked by the therapist. When Mr. Smith smokes, the therapist smokes. When he strips off his coat, the therapist removes his coat. The therapist points out that they are the same age. They are both workers. The therapist too is restless.

These mimetic responses jolt Mr. Smith out of his position as the deviant. Because the therapist is an expert and the most powerful member of the therapeutic system, to be like him cannot be a form of deviance. The same "twin-making" maneuvers challenge the other family members' experience. If the deviant member of their family is like the powerful therapist, then he can no longer be considered as deviant. This process starts at the very beginning of the session. When

Mr. Smith says, "I am the problem," the therapist replies, "Don't be so sure."

As the session progresses, the therapist insists that Mr. Smith is reacting to events within the family. Although this point of view is strenuously resisted, eventually it penetrates. Mr. Smith's behavior begins to be perceived as a response to the behavior of other family members. The validity of the family experience is again challenged.

Late in the session, the therapist develops the strategy of making Mrs. Smith the patient. Because this view is directly contrary to the family's experience of Mr. Smith as the deviant, it is resisted. However, Mrs. Smith accepts the label of being sick because it holds out the promise of meeting her needs, which until now have been subordinated to Mr. Smith's needs. The previous complementarity is reversed. Mrs. Smith, the victimized, sacrificing helper of the deviant Mr. Smith, now becomes the patient. The previously identified patient is required to help the new deviant.

At the same time, Mr. Smith's centrality within the system is preserved. This position is clearly important both to him and to his family. But aspects of his personality that have fallen into disuse can now emerge, so he can become the helper instead of the helped.

The strategy works, and its success is made possible by several factors. The therapist has directly supported Mr. Smith. Because Mr. Smith feels confirmed by an alliance with the therapist, it becomes valuable to him. To maintain this alliance, Mr. Smith must accept the reality of his wife's needs and perceive himself as helping her rather than as always receiving help from her. This shift jars the family out of its groove. Mr. Smith's experience, as the product of internal and external factors, changes. He is no longer seen as a deviant, but as the therapist's "twin." He is no longer regarded as the helped, but the helper. This transformation of the family structure makes it possible for hitherto submerged transactional patterns to emerge. These new patterns, in addition to being self-supporting, will be reinforced in therapy.

Following this session, a discussion is held with Dr. Farrell about strategies for continuing to work with the couple. When Dr. Farrell decides that she does not have enough background in family therapy to work with the couple, the case is referred to a family therapist, Mariano Barragan, M.D. He meets with the couple about twenty times over a ten-month period. The focus shifts to Mrs. Smith and the couple's sexual problems, and techniques like those developed by Masters and Johnson are brought in.[1] The therapist also helps the family to establish a more defined life space for Mr. Brown, apart from the couple. The grandfather begins to go out to visit friends more, and he makes a point of retiring to his part of the house during the evenings. The case is terminated by mutual agreement. A follow-up three years later indicates that Mr. Smith is still competently employed at the same job, and the family is functioning harmoniously. In this case, a family-oriented intervention has avoided hospitalization.

10 A "Yes, And" Technique: The Dodds and Carl A. Whitaker

The Dodds family was seen by Carl A. Whitaker as a demonstration in family interviewing after they had been in treatment for over a month with a family therapy team composed of a psychologist and a social work student on the staff of the Philadelphia Child Guidance Clinic. The session transcribed here has the problems inherent in demonstrations. The interviewer will not have contact with the family or the therapists again. He is relating to two audiences—the family requiring treatment and the professional audience being taught. His interventions are directed to both contexts and goals. However, the demonstration interview has the advantage of eliciting some of the most important characteristics of an interviewer's style.

Carl Whitaker challenges the Dodds family and seeks leverage for changing it by positing an expanded reality as available within each member. He supports the family members' responses to circumstances, conveying a sense of respect for their attempts to cope. He joins the family, dwelling on positives and potentials. Mr. and Mrs. Dodds respond to this "very nice man," as they described him a year and a half later, with an increase in self-respect and in their respect for each other. From this position, Whitaker suggests not change but self-expansion; not because the other needs it, but because it will feel good for oneself. For instance, Mr. Dodds describes himself as soft and quiet. Whitaker says, "Does your wife get scared when you really

189

come on strong?" To the wife, he says, "When he comes on strong, you come on soft. You take his line when he takes your line."

The identified patient is a quiet, frightened boy of eleven, dominated by a controlling mother. Continuing his exploration of the possibilities of experiencing in oneself the feelings one attributes to other family members with whom one is complementarily joined, Whitaker asks, "Do you ever beat her at cards? How does she take it? Does she get hurt?" Later, he asks, "Did you ever think of being your own mother's mother? You never have? Oh, it's great!"

Whitaker does not directly challenge the proximity of mother and son. Instead, he tries to change the synapses of interpersonal transactions by expanding the participants' sense of self. Structurally, he increases the proximity of husband and wife by supporting their transactions, thereby separating the mother and son and making the mother less central. With this strategy, the experience of the family members can change.

The following interview shows an interesting technique of "changing Alice's room." Whitaker begins to experience himself as being too powerful in the session. Accordingly, he moves down to the floor. When he appears low and small, the rest of the people are elevated and become more powerful. His change in position and his playing with the baby make it possible for a friendly, supportive atmosphere to develop in a family that is ordinarily tightly controlled and guilt-ridden.

Only the first twenty minutes of the interview are presented. As it begins, the psychologist is briefing Dr. Whitaker. The younger children are also present: nine-year-old Cathy, seven-year-old David, and the baby. The participants are seated as follows:

Mrs. Dodds	Mr. Dodds (giving baby a bottle)
Wise (clinic therapist)	Cathy
David	Schwartz (clinic therapist)
Whitaker	Jason

The observers are watching from behind a one-way mirror and by video monitor, so that their presence does not intrude.

Schwartz: . . . wetting problem with Jason which the family felt kind of divided about. Mrs. Dodds felt that it was a real problem. Mr. Dodds seemed to be more patient about it, felt that it was something that would go away.

Whitaker: Is there anything you want to add to this? To what he was saying?

Re. Directs question to the whole family.

Mrs. Dodds: Well, it's very hard to cover a situation where we've been talking for weeks with the therapists. I guess that through these sessions I have found that I am expecting too much out of my first-born, out of the older one. I expect him to assume responsibilities that I don't really feel are too mature for an eleven-year-old, going on his age at this point. I don't think that requiring things of him within reason is expecting too much, such as taking dirty clothes out of his room and putting them in the hamper. And at night—because I don't make the bed every morning for the mere fact that it's wet. So I say, "Jason, you are very capable. There are plenty of clean sheets. You can put one on." At night, after the bed is dried a little, I go in. I have a deodorant that I use in the room because he's a big boy. You know, I am trying to eliminate the possibility of odor.

Whitaker: Does he object to the odor, or does it just bother you?

Ac. Follows the content.
Re. A message about individuation is implied.

Mrs. Dodds: Well, it bothers me because I certainly don't want that odor in the home. And with boys this age it—if it's not taken care of to a degree—I don't know if you are too familiar with it, but Doctor, it does happen. I have walked into other homes where the place just reeked of urine, and I think, "Oh, my," you know.

Whitaker: Is it just the urine odor that bothers you, or are there other odors that bother you too?

Ac. The therapist follows the content and keeps contact with the mother, who has defined herself as the family switchboard and engaged the therapist. *Re.* Instead of focusing on the child's problem, the therapist asks what bothers the mother, regarding her as a patient.

Mrs. Dodds: Well, I guess you have odor—garlic—around the house, and you don't want it to be too strong.

Whitaker: No, I mean about him.

Mrs. Dodds: Oh, no. We make him wash.

Whitaker: You sounded as though there was somebody on the other side. Is it just Jason on the other side, or is Dad sort of opposed to this effort of yours to get rid of the odor?

Ac. Tracking (following content) and structure maintenance (talking with the switchboard).
Re. Explores the possibility of a coalition of the father and son against the mother.

Mrs. Dodds: No, no, he—I do this entirely on my own. I don't think Jack, half the time, is aware in the daytime how I holler about, "Get those wet sheets off the bed! Throw them in the hamper!" And every day the hamper is collected, and every day I wash. I mean, I'm not the cleanest person in the world. My home, if you walk into it this morning, Doctor, you may have to climb over a toy, or, you know, or the kids' things are on the floor and my dining room needs a wiping up. But—

Whitaker (to Wise): Would you do me a favor? Change places with Jason? *(Jason and the therapist change, so Jason is now between David and his mother.)*

Re. Changes a seating arrangement that had put Jason outside the family.

Mrs. Dodds: About the children's health habits, I guess I am a little bit sensitive. Especially that I know that he wets. And he is getting to be a big boy, and in the morning he must wash and everything is clean and dry in the morning. I make sure that he washes— well, you don't want to go to school smelling. Because I have had the experience with—other children would come near me, and they just reeked, like they didn't bother. And he, at times, if he can get away with it, if I don't get after him, he sometimes for- gets. And he'll come by me, and I'll say, "You didn't change." Or, "You didn't wash good enough." And this is like in the morning before he goes to school—

Whitaker: You sound like there is fire in your eyes when you say that.

Ac. Although criticizing how the mother talks about her son, he does so in such a way as not to imply criticism of her as a person. The statement could be a compliment to her vitality.

Mrs. Dodds: —and I think, "You're not going to school like that."

Whitaker: There is, huh?

Mrs. Dodds: We may not be the best dressers, or anything, but let's be a little clean. Soap don't cost that much. But it's very difficult. I think that he should be able to do this. Get the dirty wash out of his room and put it in the hamper.

Whitaker: You started to say some- thing, Dad.

Ac. Responds to a gesture from the father, to establish contact with him.

Mr. Dodds: He also had a problem of messing himself. Which seems to be pretty good in the last few months.

Whitaker: Tell me how you feel about your therapist team?

Re. Reminds the father and the others that he is in a consultant's role. He wants to effect a clear disengagement from the other therapists, so as to follow a line of exploration that deals more with growth and possibilities and less with pathology.

Mr. Dodds: Oh, seem to be doing a fine job.

Whitaker: You work well with them? You feel quite comfortable with them?

Mr. Dodds: Yes, quite comfortable. He also had an aversion to using toilet paper. Why, I don't know. He would pick up anything he could find in the hamper to wipe himself. Why he had an aversion to toilet paper, I don't know. This was another problem that used to bother us.

Whitaker: Maybe he's worried about his fingers going through it. How's about it? You getting along with the family better since the business up here? (*Jason looks at his mother.*)

Re. Suggests a logical reason for the child's behavior instead of regarding it as crazy. The therapist uses the father's statement as a bridge for making direct contact with the identified patient, who has only been talked about. His question is related to interpersonal transactions between the identified patient and the family; it does not inquire into pathology.

Mrs. Dodds: He's talking to you, Jason.

Whitaker: Do you like coming up here or is it a pain in the neck? (*Jason shrugs.*) You look all dressed up today. Do you always dress up like that? (*Jason shakes his head.*) You look like a seventeen-year-old.

Ac. and *Re.* Talks with the identified patient, who has been described as smelly and ill-groomed, commenting on his good appearance and seeming maturity.

Mrs. Dodds: Do you go to school, Jason? Don't you get dressed like this every morning?

Jason: Yeah.

Mrs. Dodds: Well, why did you say no? This is his school clothes because we are ready to let them go right back. That's why I let Cathy wear her uniform.

Whitaker: You look most dignified. I wish I could get my eleven-year-old dressed up like that.

Re. Refuses mother's bid to continue making contact with the therapist for the entire family.

Ac. Maintains contact with the identified patient, making him a model. He also identifies himself as the father of a child of the same age who is disobedient.

Mr. Dodds: He doesn't look like that when he comes home, though.

Mrs. Dodds: He looks like that going out, but not coming home.

Whitaker: Thank heaven for that.

Re. Reinforces the message that a lack of order is normal. The therapist's tone is casual, and he addresses no one in particular. Nevertheless, this statement is one of a series that conveys his value system to the family.

Mrs. Dodds: He is required in school to wear a white shirt and jacket every day, so that each morning they are clean-looking going out the door. That's his school clothes. Well, the pants are new, but—

Whitaker: You just starting your long pants?

Ac. Uses the mother's statement as a bridge to make contact with another member without rejecting her.

Mrs. Dodds: He's talking to you, David.

Whitaker: How long ago?

Mrs. Dodds: Answer the gentleman, David.

Whitaker: It's awful early to wear long pants. I thought kids were—you wear slacks when you're what? What are you? Ten?

Ac. Though the content reveals only the therapist's ignorance of changing children's styles, his intention of establishing a dialog with the child is clear.

Mr. Dodds: Can't you talk? Talk to the doctor.

Schwartz: You know, this is the first time that David and I have met. It's the first time that I've seen you here. And I'm struck about how similar David and Jason are about the business of answering questions. I

Ac. Schwartz provides a bridge between the previous therapeutic system and the consultant. Schwartz's style, quite different from Whitaker's, deals with pathology and resistance.

think one of the experiences we have had with Jason being here is it's been hard for us to talk together at times. And we're not sure why that is. Sometimes Mrs. Dodds comes in and answers questions.

Whitaker: It sounds to me like there is enough fire in Mom's voice so that it must make him kind of hesitate, huh?

Re. Explains the child's behavior in terms of his interaction with the mother. The repeated metaphor is not negative, for it does not allude to the mother's control or anger. The imagery suggests a goddess, who could inspire fear, respect, or adoration, as well as hesitation.

The mother feels challenged and accommodates to the therapist.

Mrs. Dodds: No, I haven't prompted them in any way because I don't know what questions you'll ask. My only words were—Jason, tell Dr. Whitaker what I told you in the event that you are asked a question.

Jason: What?

Mrs. Dodds: When I told you at home, whatever you are asked—what did I tell you?

Cathy: To answer it.

Mrs. Dodds: To what, Cathy? To answer it. This is the only prompting that I gave them. If there's any question asked, no matter what it is, answer it.

Whitaker: Come on, Dad. Do you solve the problem of Mom coming on so strong by sort of being nice and quiet?

Re. Contacts the father, avoiding answering the mother directly and having to challenge her. The therapist makes an interpretation of complementarity in the husband-wife relationship. Again, the terms emphasize positives: the mother is strong, the father is nice. Another therapist, more concerned with pathology, might call her controlling and him passive.

Mr. Dodds: Yes, I think we are quite opposite in personality. She is, like you say, quite fiery.

Whitaker: Do you appreciate that? Do you like it?

Mr. Dodds: Yes, I guess in a way it's good.

Whitaker: I sort of feel like that's the way we marry. I married a wife with fire because I was kind of soft and easy.

Ac. Both spouses and their transactional patterns are supported. The spouse subsystem boundary is defined, which protects both spouses. The mother is not isolated as the controlling switchboard, as she started in the session, and the father is not isolated as the nurturer (he has been silent since feeding the baby). Increasing the active proximity of the spouses will also free the identified patient from the mother's hovering attention. The therapist's mimesis also supports husband and wife, showing he is like them.

Re. Talking with the father makes him more central, reducing the mother's turf.

Mr. Dodds: And she's like the life of the party.

Whitaker: No, I think I gained a lot from her fire. And I suspect it's the other way around. That she married you in the hopes of quieting down some of her fire.

Ac. Mimesis increases his accommodation to the family. The therapist and father become twins through a similar experience.

Re. Sends an indirect message to the mother suggesting change ("quieting down some of her fire"), as though it came from her. This reinforces the spouse subsystem boundary by assigning to the husband the function of actively helping his wife.

Mr. Dodds: I kind of think it's a balancing effect. It's nice.

Whitaker: I have often had the fantasy of, if two fireballs like your wife were to get married, the place would go up in smoke. And if two soft guys like you or like me were to get married, we'd end up blah, blah, blah.

Mrs. Dodd: That, I agree. I often say that. My goodness, what would happen if he ever married a girl like himself? No fun, Hon'!

Mr. Dodds: That's true. I think maybe that's why you get together.

Whitaker (to baby): Hello. Do you want to come and see me? Come on, come on. (*He puts baby on his lap.*) How's that? Do you want to get down? (*Baby gets down.*)

Mrs. Dodds: He's a very friendly child.

Whitaker: Wonderful smile. Bye. (*Baby crawls to the mother.*)

Mrs. Dodds: Here, show the man how you can stand up pretty good already. No jumping.

Whitaker: That's great. You want to walk over to my finger? Come on. (*He gets down on floor and holds arms out to the baby.*)

Ac. The therapist joins the family in its nurturant aspect by picking up the baby, who has been wandering around to various family members to be picked up.

Ac. De-emphasizes formality. The action also requests a family accommodation to the therapist and his expressed value system—nurturance, relaxation, acceptance of diversity, and a soft, easy-going style.
Re. Implicitly supports the father, who, as the therapist's twin, also becomes "soft but strong."
An alternative transactional pattern now appears in response to the therapist's behavior. The mother is softer, almost seductive, and a general mood of pride and contentment, with the baby at the center, appears.

Mrs. Dodds (The baby crawls back to her): Did you decide you wanted your mother? Okay then, come on. You want to stand right there and say hello to the doctor? He's a very nice man, isn't he?

Cathy: Hey! (*She takes the baby.*)

Whitaker (still on the floor): Do the boys ever get on fire like Momma? Or do they pretty much stay like you?

Mr. Dodds: I don't know. They are pretty even-dispositioned. At times they blow up.

Whitaker: Do you blow up at times too?

Re. Continues to centralize the father, weaving in his modeling for his children.

Ac. Tracking. Exploring an aspect of the father's behavior confirms him.

Mr. Dodds: Sometimes.

Whitaker: How does it go?

Mr. Dodds: Very seldom. It would have to be an issue that's built up for a long time before I really blow up.

Whitaker: Does Momma get scared when you really come on strong?

Re. Presents the possibility of "frightening" behavior in the family member whose identity in the family has been styled soft and quiet. The therapist expands the boundaries of possible individual alternatives, a technique he will use later on.

Mr. Dodds: Nah! (*Both parents laugh.*)

Mrs. Dodds: I don't mean to laugh, but really, Jack doesn't come on where I've ever been afraid of him. He'll holler, and I let him. When he's blowing up, I just let him holler.

Whitaker: You take his line when he takes your line. When he comes on strong, you come on soft.

Ac. An educational input.
Re. Emphasizes the complementarity of husband-wife behavior.

Mrs. Dodds: Well, if I think he is absolutely wrong, or—gee, I can't even remember what we argued about, really, that would be serious. He may holler about something, and I will think, oh, well, let him go on, and I just don't answer him. And if there is an issue that is very important, it seems like where I would tend to become very upset about it, we wait until after the children are in bed. We will discuss whatever—say there has to be an important decision. We don't discuss everything in front of the children, but there's not too much that we don't. But there are some things that we must make a decision on, and we don't discuss it in front of the children.

Whitaker: Do you ever think that keeps them—if they don't see you fight—

Ac. Continues contact with the mother, who has defined herself as the central member.
Re. Introduces a different value—the importance to child development for children to see parents fighting, disagreeing, or handling conflict.

Mrs. Dodds: In most—oh no, we don't hide. Like, an important decision with the thing that we can or cannot afford, it involves the children. The situation arises, right then and there it's settled. I mean, Jason isn't unaware that Jack and I may argue a point. But, like any big decisions, when I make, I might get very nervous—we discuss this quietly because Jack is the quiet kind. I'll say, "Now look. Let's just look at this thing."

Whitaker: When you get nervous, he becomes your therapist somehow.

Re. Again emphasizes spouse complementarity.

Mrs. Dodds: Well, I think so. Because I do respect the fact that he thinks things out long and hard before he would make a decision, to say "yes" or "no" to something that I wanted to do. Like, we had discussed coming here previously, and we looked at both sides. We looked at the fact that we will have to give time. We've tried to do—you know, like a few times we've had to miss because of sickness. But when we made up our mind we were coming, we made up our mind together that we would *both*—that Daddy is going to come if he is requested. He comes. And this is a lot for the working man, to run home and run here. And he could be very well sitting at home. But he said, "No, Hon', I'll go all the way."

Whitaker (tickling the baby): And if he ever gets around to really saying "no," will you then buckle him under?

Mrs. Dodds: No. If after he points out what he feels is nothing, not the right thing, I usually go by his judgment. There is not too many instances where this happens. Jack more or less gives me the freedom. He feels I'm in the home all day, and I am the one that has to live with certain things. I mean, you can't be too specific, Doctor, because I would have to—

Whitaker: No, that's all right. Do you ever get the sense that this is quite a burden, this carrying it all on your shoulders?

Re. Relabels, introducing an idea he will develop later—the wife's "duty" (her overcontrolling) as burdensome. *Ac.* Shows sympathy and respect, by relabeling in the form of a concerned question.

Mrs. Dodd (hesitates): No, I don't feel that it's a burden. I don't feel that I'm always doing the best thing, you know?

Whitaker: Of course, don't we all? It's one of the things about being a parent.

Ac. This message, "we are all more human than otherwise" (as H.S. Sullivan put it), threads through many of the therapist's comments. It is part of his humanistic, normalizing message.

Mrs. Dodds: I worry about Jason, and I don't know why, because he's never been in any kind of trouble. He's a nice kid. We have lots of fun around the house in playing games, or—what games do we play? (*To Jason.*) Monopoly? He's a little sore loser. I beat him at 500 rummy, or something, and—

Whitaker: Do you ever beat her?

Re. Again offers a family member an expansion of possible behavior. The word "beat" is used with both meanings—winning and thrashing. The therapist's operation with Jason, a quiet boy, is similar to that with the father.
Ac. Confirms the identified patient as a competent observer of the mother's behavior.

Jason (laughs): Sometimes.

Whitaker: Really? How does she take it? She get hurt?

Mrs. Dodds: Look at the doctor.
Whitaker: Take it out on you later?
Jason: No. (*He laughs.*)
Whitaker: No?
Mrs. Dodds (To Whitaker): Oh, no.
Whitaker: Is she proud of you when you beat her?

Re. Again expands the boundaries of the "acceptable me," introducing possible vistas of behavior that the identified patient has not even imagined—that the mother might accept him and even be proud of him if he beat her.

Jason: No.
Whitaker: I remember the first time my son gave me a black eye.

Ac. Talks of his own experience as a father. Here the ambiguous "beating" clearly takes on a violent meaning.

Mrs. Dodds: I'm talking about cards.
Whitaker: I was mad as the dickens at him, but I was kind of tickled. You know—the son of a gun.

Ac. Models normal behavior, feeling mad but proud. Having first declared himself the father's twin, and now the mother's twin, the therapist proclaims his own feeling and suggests this possibility for his "twins."

Mrs. Dodds: Well, this is only in games of cards. He doesn't hit me yet. I'm saying "yet," because sometimes I think when I'm after him for something he—only the fact that I'm his mother, you know, holds his hands down. Because he gets very ired at me.
Whitaker: So you're like your pop. You just blow your stack once in a while. What do you think would happen—(*pauses to tickle the baby*)—what do you think would happen if you won an argument with Mother and proved she was wrong?

Re. Frames the son's behavior in response to his mother as similar to the father's. The therapist talks to the son and sends a message to the father.

Jason: I don't know.
Whitaker: Suppose you caught her? You know, you really caught her? (*He tickles the baby.*)
Mrs. Dodds: Tell him what you think, Jason.

Whitaker: Do you think she would cry? Did you ever see her cry?

Re. Again expands the experience of other family members. At the beginning of the session, the therapist asked the mother to see her son as a dignified "seventeen-year-old," better than the therapist's son. Now he asks the son to see his powerful mother as weak.

Jason: Sometimes.

Whitaker: Good. Were you her mommy then? Did you ever think of being your own mother's mother? You know, if she gets real nervous and upset and feels like crying, do you come over and cuddle her and make her feel better? Do you ever do that?

Re. Playing the metaphor of being "your mother's mother" challenges the boy to see himself as a mother. The therapist has asked the family members to think and feel like each other in a play of expanding images.

Jason: Nope.

Whitaker: You never have? Oh, it's great. I came home one day from the office, and I was feeling lousy and lay down on the couch and shut my eyes and asked the kids if they would just leave me alone. And after I had been laying there for a few minutes, my little six-year-old came over and gave me a kiss. You know, my headache went away just like magic.

Ac. Moves back to be like the family, now as a parent experiencing his child's behavior. The therapist then requests that the family accommodate to his way of experiencing.

Mrs. Dodds: Don't look at me and laugh, Jason. That's simple, now. Look at the doctor. He's speaking to you.

The mother may feel embarrassed for being what she is instead of being like the therapist. She attacks her son.

Whitaker: Maybe he never thought about being his mother's mother. Do they get the sense that you're ashamed when you get nervous and upset? That you're embarrassed—embarrassed about being nervous, when you get nervous?

Ac. Responds to her discomfort with support and an insightful leap into her feelings.

Mrs. Dodd: I don't think so.

Whitaker: Are you embarrassed—sort of ashamed to be weak?

Re. Helps the mother expose herself as weak to her family, especially to Jason.

Mrs. Dodd: Well, I get mad at myself for blowing. Sometimes for, you know—it seems like I more get mad at

myself than ashamed. Let's put it
that way. I'm not ashamed that I have
hollered at them or that I have an
emotion. It's just that I don't know
how to cope with a situation, then I
get mad at myself. Yeah, for having
blown up that minute, and I should
have just waited until his father came
home, or something—

Whitaker: You feel you ought to be
more—

Mrs. Dodds: —but I've never believed
in carrying over a problem until the
father comes home, because either you
forget the problem or the kid forgets
what he's getting hollered at for. In
that sense—

Whitaker: Good for you.

Mrs. Dodds: So I end up with most
of the disciplining.

Whitaker: How about when you
apologize? Do you apologize? Tell him
you're wrong?

Mrs. Dodds: Oh, yes, I have had the
occasion. Haven't I, Jason? (*Jason
laughs.*) Apologize to you. Haven't I
said, "Well, I'm sorry, Jason, I—"
Let's see. It wasn't too long ago that I
said—that I found out later I was wrong.

Jason (laughs): When was that?

Mrs. Dodds: How about when I took
you to school the other day, and I said
that I was sorry that we pushed you so
hard, not knowing what was going on
in school. Didn't I say that? Not knowing the pressures you were under.

Whitaker: Does he forgive you all
right, then?

Ac. Supports.

Re. Educates. The therapist's values
about being human guide some of his
questions. A significant value for him
is the ability of people to confirm and
recognize other people.

*The session started with a central, con-
trolling mother who was always right,
complaining about a disappointing
son. The therapist's intervention has
moved the mother-son transactional
patterns to a possible alternative
pattern, in which an embarrassed,
guilty mother is apologizing to her son.
Re. Again switches the identified
patient from one who is incompetent
to one who has the power to forgive or
not forgive a guilty mother.*

Mrs. Dodds: Do you forgive me, Jason?

Jason (laughs): Yeah.

Mr. Dodds: He's not very compassionate. Like, if he gets his mother riled to the point where she'll break down or cry or something—

Whitaker: He kind of enjoys it, huh?

Mr. Dodds: I don't say he enjoys it, but he don't come over and try to make up or anything like this. Yet at times when everything is fine, he'll come over and give his mother a kiss or a hug or something.

Mrs. Dodds: Oh, yeah.

Whitaker: I just had a crazy thought. Do you like crazy thoughts? I love my crazy thoughts. They are more fun than the usual ones. The crazy thought I had was that he was trying to teach you how to handle your wife. Maybe you are too forgiving.

Re. Breaking boundaries of separation and individual roles, the therapist suggests that the father can learn from his son.

11 The Initial Interview: The Gordens and Braulio Montalvo

The goals of a family interview are one of the factors that help to define how the therapist will conduct the session. The interviews with the Wagners and the Rabins were explorations of effective family functioning. The interviewers' inputs were confined largely to accommodation and diagnostic probes. With the Smith and Dodds families, the therapists were consultants. The Smiths were just entering family therapy, and the Dodds had been in family therapy for some months, but both therapists knew they would not be continuing with the families. This interview with the Gorden family is the first transcript of the initial contact of a family with a therapist who is planning to go on with that family in therapy.

An initial session has the unique characteristics of a meeting between two social units of strangers. Therefore, at first it takes on the form of a social gathering. There may be many hesitations, trials, and tentative searches for the right level of contact. The therapist's chief concern is to develop the therapeutic unit. But he must also begin to map the family structure, broaden the focus (if the presenting problem has been an individual family member), and most important, develop at least an interim therapeutic contract.

There are other tasks that the family therapist must perform in all sessions, but which assume special form during the initial session. At the beginning of the session the therapist must act as the family's host. He must also be careful to make contact with all family members.

Thus, an initial session can tentatively be divided into three stages.

In the first stage, the therapist follows the cultural rules of etiquette. In the second stage, he asks each member of the family what he thinks are the problems in the family. In the third stage, he explores the family structure by helping the family enact their family drama. Of course, these stages are subject to variation and modification by an experienced family therapist.

THE FAMILY THERAPIST AS HOST

The opening contact with a family can be viewed as a host-guest relationship. The family is ill at ease. They do not know the rules of the game, and they do not know the therapist, except that they presume he is an expert who will help them with their problem as they perceive it. They are on the therapist's turf. They expect that he, as the host, will establish the rules by which they are to relate to him.

The therapist's first concern is to put the family at ease. He introduces himself and helps the family introduce themselves to him. If he has gotten their names from a telephone conversation or the brief notes of an intake secretary, he matches the names to each family member. This shows that he has prepared for the family. If possible, he should have equipped the room before the family's arrival with enough chairs. If there are small children, he may wish to provide small chairs and some quiet toys.

When the family sits down, the family therapist should pay attention to how they position themselves. Often their placement can give him some hunches about family affiliations. This is minimal data, to which the family therapist should not give too much weight. Nevertheless, it does sometimes provide clues that can later be tested.

The therapist may spend the first few minutes in small talk. If there is special equipment in use, such as audio or video recorders, he should explain it. He may ask the family if they had a difficult time coming. This is living room behavior, conforming to cultural rules of politeness.

MAKING THERAPEUTIC CONTACTS

As soon as the therapist discerns that the family is feeling more comfortable, he asks what problem has brought the family into the session. This question frames the nature of the task that has drawn together an expert helper and a family in need. The response of the family is in itself an indication of how the family negotiates boundaries with the outside world and of what the family wants to project as an image.

At this point the family is in an artificial environment, meeting a therapist who is a stranger. Therefore, they will behave in "official" ways. A family with tenuous boundaries with the outside world may begin to include the therapist in their conflicts and fights immediately. Other families will protect themselves by giving an official version of their family, opening up to the therapist only after he has joined them in a therapeutic system.

The therapist's first question is usually posed in generic terms and not clearly directed to any family member in particular. For example, he may say, "Well, let's find out what has brought you here." But the therapist can also decide to address this question to a specific member. If the parents are sitting together, he can direct his question to them by looking in their direction.

Sometimes the first question is determined by the family's cultural values or by a shared value system. For example, a male therapist may speak first to the father because of a common value system. Or it may be useful to speak first to the father for other reasons. For example, when working with a poor family, the therapist assumes that the mother has been given the responsibility and obligation of parenting and connecting with agencies, for she is automatically considered to be more knowledgeable about a child's problem and more skilled in making contact with agencies. However, if the therapist directs his first question to the mother, the father may disengage. An initial question addressed to the father will send the message that the therapist considers him a significant person within the family who should participate. Even if the father then refers the question to his wife, he has now been contacted. His referring of the question is itself a form of participation.

Next, the therapist begins to spread his contact. In an intact family, he begins to draw in the other spouse. If the mother has presented the problem, the therapist then asks the father what his view of the situation is. If the father has spoken, the therapist addresses the mother.

He pays special attention to the similarities and differences in the way each parent presents the problems. For example, the mother may emphasize the disobedience of a child, but the father may qualify this by saying that the child is very disobedient with his wife. The nature of the qualification, or even an inflection of voice, may cue the therapist to explore this area. When he probes, the father may say that the child obeys him, but his wife is too lenient. Now, very quickly, the therapist finds himself in the middle of an interspouse conflict. The problem explicitly defined by the parents five minutes before was the child's disobedience. Already this has broadened to an area of disagreement between the parents.

The therapist's next move depends on his assessment of the family. He may allow or even encourage the parental conflict to develop as a strategy for moving the "problem" label away from the child and exploring a possibly dysfunctional husband-wife subsystem. However, he must be careful not to open up areas of stress before the therapeutic system has developed to a point where he can support the family members under stress. If such interspouse conflict comes too early in the first session, the therapist may merely have to register it as an area for future exploration and disarm the issue by moving to another family member.

The therapist listens to the content of the family's presentation of the problem, but he also looks at the way in which the family behaves. On a nonverbal level, they are probably much less constrained, and their behavior is probably more similar to its accustomed pattern. The therapist notices nonverbal communications between the children and the parents. If the children are restless, do they move around or do they check with mother first? If one parent begins to talk, does the other interrupt to qualify or negate what is being said? When one family member is talking, do the others listen to what he is saying? What are the signals by which family members cue each other as to what is an acceptable communication in the context of the session? The family therapist will ultimately need to know how the family transacts and how it responds to situations of stress within the family. Observing it on a nonverbal level is a first step toward this understanding.

After the family therapist has elicited the parents' presentation of the problem, he will ask a third member for his opinion. That person should not, in general, be the identified patient, for if the parents have focused on one child as the problem, that child is in a defensive position. If the therapist contacts him, he may then feel that the therapist is joining and accepting the coalition which puts the blame on him. Contacting another family member first may allow for the appearance of a different slant on the problem, opening a new area of family problems.

The therapist should at some point relate to each of the family members present, including the youngest children. A very young child may not be asked to present his view of the problem, but the therapist can exchange some words or affectionate gestures with him so as to make him feel that he is a part of the session.

It is not essential for each member of the family to be contacted sequentially, with the therapist not proceeding further until each person has been contacted. But it is important, in the first session, that each member feel he has participated with the therapist in the exploration of problems.

EXPLORING FAMILY STRUCTURE

Up to this point, the family members will have addressed themselves largely to the family therapist, the expert. He has been eliciting their comments in a fishing expedition. He listens to what they say, but his chief concern is trying to understand the way the family functions. He begins to get an idea of the family structure by observing the sequences in which people talk. He looks at how the family members relate to each other. Does the mother act as a switchboard, all communication passing through her? Does the father interrupt her, talking louder than she does? Does a dyadic interaction develop? Does it escalate? Are dyadic interactions diffused by the inclusion of another member?

At the same time the therapist is planning his next moves. He is thinking of strategies most likely to be effective in making the family reveal itself. Up to now, the family has presented a rehearsed communication to a person who has accepted their communication without challenge. The therapist has probably been the most active member of the session; he has at least been the instrumental leader of the session in the sense of having directed communication, asking first one member and then another to talk.

He has been mapping certain aspects of the family structure and has been generous with joining maneuvers. Now he feels that his interventions are no longer random. He has hunches, which he wants to test. His position with the family has been strengthened by his careful transactions with its members in accordance with their family structure. As a result, stressful interventions can be accepted as coming from a member of the therapeutic system.

So far, the family therapist has responded to the family's expectation that the expert to whom they have come for assistance will indicate how they should describe a problem to him. Now he must change that set. He must give the ball back to the family and observe how they handle a situation in their own terms. If this is not accomplished, he will be unable to observe the larger field of the family pattern. Therefore, he begins to organize the family into subsystems and to probe with more freedom, guided by his assessment of the family. If he has observed areas of disagreement between husband and wife, he can begin to probe by directing the spouses to talk to each other. Or if there is a problem between mother and child, he can activate that dyad.

When the members of the subsystem selected are talking to each other and transacting negotiations, the family therapist can use a wide lens; he does not have to intervene. The family is operating with increased intensity of affect because the situation is one that usually exists at home. If the mother and father are discussing differences with regard to the children, the family therapist is observing the parental dyad and the response of the other family members to a parental dyad transaction.

At this point the family therapist functions very much like the director of a play. By directing certain members to talk with one another, he is testing his hunches about the way in which the family functions. He probes areas of disagreement and observes how disagreement is handled and how the family resolves a problem. He is also gathering information for his next strategy, which may be to include another member in the ongoing negotiation or to explore a different dyad.

The family therapist is guided, in this initial exploration, by his idea of an effectively functioning family. He is looking for the qualities of differentiation, delineation of boundaries, and flexibility. But at the same time, he is looking for dysfunctional sets.

BROADENING THE FOCUS

The technique of organizing the family into subsystems also helps to broaden the focus of the problem. Usually the family has come into therapy with one identified patient. Their goals and the therapist's are not the same. The family has organized itself to focus on the identified patient and is sometimes very concerned with maintaining that focus. The family therapist, by contrast, assumes from the start that the identified patient is responding to dysfunctional aspects of family transactions, and that the best way to approach the problems of the identified patient is through highlighting and changing those dysfunctional aspects. Often the initial session oscillates between these two viewpoints. The family therapist expands the focus of exploration from the identified patient to different aspects of the family organization; the family swings the problem back to focus on the identified patient. The therapist presents the need to explore the way the family operates and offers means to do so. The family may hear the message and sometimes even respond to it, but later they narrow the focus again, pointing toward the identified patient.

The family therapist may use many strategies to broaden the focus. He can select another patient on whom to concentrate. He can discuss other problems. He can explore related areas. For example, if a child is presented as having problems in school, he can ask if the child has problems at home. If a problem at home is brought up, it can be discussed in terms of interpersonal transactions.

The exploration of dyads may be helpful. If there is a problem between parent and parent, the problems between parent and child or between child and child can be opened up for exploration. It is useful to look for positives in the identified patient and urge the family to acknowledge them.

If the session has been conducted well, the family and the therapist will probably reach agreement that it is necessary to explore beyond the identified patient. This conclusion may be stressful for the family, but it also offers an element of hope. The family has come to therapy because of its failure to solve the problem with the identified patient. By expanding the problem beyond the family focus, the therapist raises the hope that a different way of looking at the problem will bring a solution.

In many ways the initial interview is an encapsulation of what will happen with the family in therapy. Points of stress must be explored, but the family therapist must be aware of the level of stress that the family can tolerate. When family members become too uncomfortable, the therapist must move back, often by using maintenance operations, to a point where the family is once again comfortable. The therapist must position himself as leader and maintain that position. Finally, all therapeutic interventions must be made with the clear knowledge that the first rule of therapeutic strategy is to leave the family willing to come again for the next session.

The idiosyncrasies of an individual family and the style of a particular family therapist are the factors that lie between the goals of a first interview and the realities of a first interview. Always, the therapist and the family must accommodate to each other in the development of a therapeutic system. Without this melding of idiosyncrasies, there will be no therapy.

The first interview that follows was conducted by an experienced family therapist, Braulio Montalvo. It follows a somewhat modified sequence. The first stage is short, the therapist's subsequent assimilation into the family system is quick, and then his contacts with all of the family members are interrupted by a strong concentration on the identified patient, seven-year-old Mandy. But all the prescribed tasks of the initial interview are achieved.

The therapist's structural assessment of the Gorden family is that it is composed of an executive subsystem, the mother and a parental child, ten-year-old Morris. The identified patient is scapegoated by this executive system (Fig. 43). The therapist's initial interventions are

Fig. 43

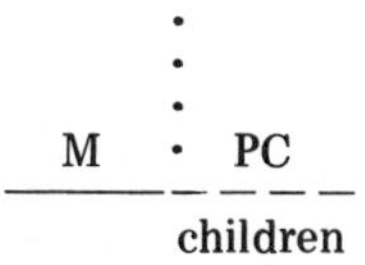

$$M \quad \cdot \quad PC$$
children

designed to affiliate with the scapegoated child and to move the parental child out of the conflict between mother and identified patient (Fig. 44).

Fig. 44

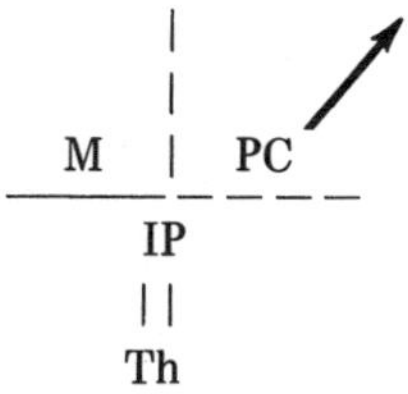

$$M \quad | \quad PC$$
IP
Th

This intervention is assimilated by the mother, and probably by the parental child, into a family structure that existed previously, before the parents separated. The mother and parental child were then in coalition against the father and identified patient, and the mother attacked the father through the identified patient (Fig. 45).

Fig. 45

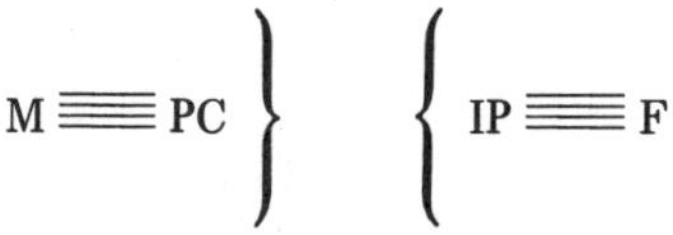

$$M \equiv PC \} \quad \{ IP \equiv F$$

The mother therefore responds to the therapist's affiliation with the identified patient by increasing her attack on the girl.

As a result, the family therapist then changes his strategy, supporting the mother in order to support the identified patient (Fig. 46).

Fig. 46

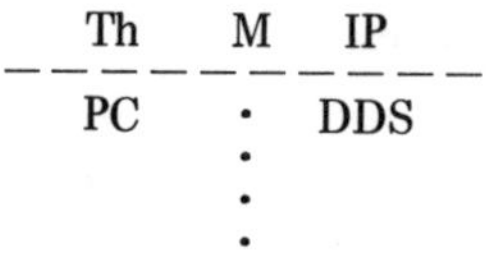

Th   M   IP
— — — — — — — —
PC   ·   DDS
      ·
      ·

He assigns a task to be performed at home that intensifies a subsystem structure in which the mother interacts directly with the identified patient, while the parental child directs his attention to his other siblings (Fig. 47). By the end of the second session, the therapist has

Fig. 47

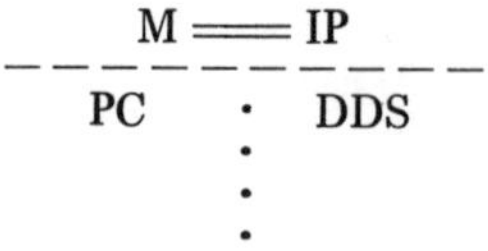

M ═══ IP
— — — — — — — —
PC   ·   DDS
      ·
      ·

begun to move toward increasing the mother's and parental child's affiliation with their extrafamilial peers (Fig. 48).

Fig. 48

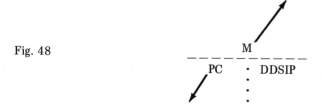

A transcript of segments of the initial interview with this family follows. The two other children in the family are also present: eight-year-old Joyce and two-year-old Debbie. When the family enters, they position themselves as follows:

Morris

Mrs. Gorden   Joyce

Debbie   Mandy

Montalvo

Montalvo: How old is she?

Ac. Contacts the mother first, acknowledging her position as executive of the family.

Mrs. Gorden: She's four.
Montalvo: Four. How old is Morris?

Ac. Knows the children's names, which suggests previous contact and accelerates entrance into the family as part of the new social system. This is living room behavior, the therapist chatting politely with the mother.

Mrs. Gorden: Ten.
Montalvo: And Annie?
Mrs. Gorden: Eight.
Montalvo: Is this Annie?

Ac. Fumbles, making a mistake first with a name, later with a child's age, which helps put the family at ease by countering any fear of absolute authority. The therapist presents himself as fallible, therefore approachable.

Mrs. Gorden: Joyce.
Montalvo: Joyce.
Mrs. Gorden: Joyce is eight.
Montalvo: Eight.
Mrs. Gorden: Mandy is seven.
Montalvo: Seven, eight, ten, and two.
Mrs. Gorden: Four.
Montalvo: Four. Boy, oh boy. Well, when you called me yesterday, you—

Ac. Refers to the only previous contact, a phone call, to give an impression of continuity and of a longer period of acquaintance.

Mrs. Gorden: I—yesterday I was so upset.
Montalvo: You were very upset.

Ac. Acknowledges and calms Mrs. Gorden's anxiety.

Mrs. Gorden: Yeah, because this could be very dangerous. And she has done it before. And if Morris had called me on the job and told me that the house was on fire again and the fire department was there, I don't know what I would have done.
Montalvo: You were on the job—

Mrs. Gorden: Yes.

Montalvo: —and Morris called you.

Mrs. Gorden: He didn't call, because he knew that I would get very upset.

Montalvo: Oh.

Mrs. Gorden: He didn't call because he had gotten it out.

Montalvo (to Morris): I see. So you handled the fire yourself?

Ac. Continues tracking the mother's communication.

Re. Contacting another member begins the teaching of a rule of communication: family members are to speak for themselves; mediation is discouraged. As Morris was there and his mother was not, this is Morris' story. This is the first tactic contrary to etiquette: the therapist interrupts Mrs. Gorden to tell Morris to talk.

Mrs. Gorden: Don't shake your head.

Mrs. Gorden challenges the therapist by correcting Morris' manners. She will insist on remaining the head of the family.

Montalvo: Who set the fire?

Morris: Mandy.

Montalvo: Mandy? Was he pretty good with the—what did you use? Water? Mandy?

Ac. Contacts a third family member. Talking with the identified patient, he seeks information; his manner is serious but not accusatory.

Mrs. Gorden: Speak up.

Montalvo: What did he use? Water?

Mandy: Yes.

Montalvo: Yeah? And what else? To put the fire out, what else did he use?

Re. Introduces second change-producing gambit. He manipulates content and affect to deal with competence—how the problem was solved— rather than who was to blame. Families in crisis tend to be concerned with identifying a culprit. Therapists must know when to challenge this behavior. Here the challenge remains implicit. The therapist models both concern for problem solving and respect for the children's competence.

Mandy: Just water.

Montalvo: Just water? He didn't throw clothing on it or anything like that?

Re. Changes the affect of a traumatic event by being interested in the description of the incident. This helps Mandy interact with him competently.

Mandy: No.

Montalvo: No. Was it really a big fire?

Ac. Asks questions in concrete fashion, so the frightened seven-year-old can answer him with monosyllables. As she begins to feel more comfortable, the questions will become more complex.

Mandy: Yes.

Montalvo: About this big? (*He holds his hands up.*) Or about this big?

Mandy: About this.

Montalvo: That big? Hoo, boy. Really something. And he did a good job.

Re. Continues using a language of competence and cooperation. This is seeding. Later in the session, he will capitalize on the exploration of this theme. At the moment, he is challenging the affect of blame. He does not confront the mother; he just suggests a different direction.

Mandy: Yes.

Montalvo: Did you help him put it out?

Mandy: No.

Montalvo: No? Did you want to help? Did you want to help to put it out? (*Mandy mumbles.*) Eh? I'm sorry, I didn't hear you.

Mrs. Gorden: Talk louder.

Mrs. Gorden accepts the therapist's acting as a facilitator. At the same time, she resumes her role as head of the family, in a controlling stance.

Mandy: He told me not to do it.

Montalvo: Can you help me understand? What did she say?

Ac. Accepts the mother's bid for leadership, using her as a translator. He follows the family's lines of communication, using the mother as the switchboard.

Re. Brings the language of support and cooperation to the dyad of mother and Mandy.

Mrs. Gorden: She said that he told her not to help. He probably told her to get out of the way.

Montalvo: Oh. Why didn't you want her to help?

Re. Again discourages the mother's talking for Morris, which reinforces the rule that family members should talk for themselves, without an intermediary.

Morris: Because she was in the way.

Montalvo: Oh? She was in the way.

Morris: 'Cause I grabbed the mattress that was on fire and I grabbed it and took it and put it in the bathroom and put it in the tub and left the water run.

Montalvo: M-hm.

Morris: And then I took all her clothes and put them in the tub.

Montalvo: You did a good job. Have you ever done anything like that before?

Ac. Rewards Morris' competence in language appropriate for a ten-year-old. He is also tracking the family's rewards for the parental child.

Re. Challenges the family's affect by concentrating its attention on positives—acts of competence.

Morris: Before, the whole thing burned. But I picked the mattress up and set it against the door, and only the mattress burned. The fire stayed small and only the mattress burned.

Mrs. Gorden: I don't even see how he did it, because I couldn't lift that mattress myself. He took the mattress off the bottom bed, and said he didn't know why he took it off. He was just excited, you know what I mean? Thinking if he got that off, the whole bed wouldn't burn up. So he started out the room with it. But he had it the long way, and it got jammed in the door. So with the mattress in the door, I don't know why he didn't get burned.

The mother's relationship to Morris emphasizes only positives, rewarding his role as parental child.

Morris: When I first came in, I just came from school. When I came in, it was only a little hole in there, and I got a whole lot of cups of water and I dumped it, but it looked like the more I dumped, the more the fire spread.

Montalvo: Mm. It started by the middle of the mattress?

Morris: M-hm.

Montalvo: Did you find out from Mandy how it got started?

Ac. Tracking.

Ac. Using content from the previously contacted member, the therapist tries to initiate a dialog between the mother and Mandy. He is enacting transactional patterns.

The mother answers the therapist instead of entering a dialog with Mandy.

Mrs. Gorden: She got some matches and lit them. She didn't say what she lit.

Montalvo: Could you ask her? Talk with her now. (*He gestures, directing Mrs. Gorden to speak directly to Mandy.*)

Ac. Maintains family structure of mother as switchboard.

Re. Directs the mother to enter a dialog with Mandy. The mother resists the therapist's intervention. He insists, wanting to see how mother and daughter interact.

The mother accommodates to the therapist, starting to talk with Mandy in an exploratory fashion. This is a good prognostic indicator of flexibility.

Mrs. Gorden: What did you do? Tell me exactly what you did when you went in my room. What did you light? When you struck the match, what did you stick it onto to make it light? How did you catch the spread on fire?

Mandy: I struck the match.

Mrs. Gorden: And just lit the spread.

The mother's tone becomes admonitory. She has reverted very quickly. Still, the prognosis is good, for Mrs. Gorden shows an ability to respond to the therapist's modeling.

Mandy: Yes.

Mrs. Gorden: You meant to light the spread?

Mandy: I was doing an experiment.

Mrs. Gorden: Well what happened? I can't hear you. You were doing an experiment?

Morris: She was—
Montalvo: Excuse me, Morris. Be-cause—go ahead, Mandy.

Re. Blocks interference by Morris, who returns to his function as the go-between between the mother and Mandy.

Mandy: I was trying—
Mrs. Gorden: With Morris' chemistry set?
Mandy: Yes! (*Mandy is crying. The therapist gestures to the mother to change seats with him. He gets up and moves toward her so she complies and sits down next to Mandy.*)

Re. Uses decrease of distance to rein-force enactment of a dialog. Before he modeled protection of Mandy; now he puts the mother in his seat, expecting his previous behavior to influence her.
The parental child explains the other children's behavior to the mother. He is following the family structure, in which he mediates between his mother and the younger children.

Morris: And then you said you wanted a drink of water. And you went out. She stayed a long time. So I went to see what she was doing. And when I got to the room, she came running in there and said, "Mommy's bed is on fire."
Montalvo: Yes. Morris is trying to be helpful, and he is. You are very help-ful. But Mandy didn't have a chance to finish her story.

Ac. Maintains a positive stance, label-ing Morris' behavior as an attempt to help.
Re. Relabels Morris' helping as in-appropriate, blocks it, and insists on the enactment of the mother-daughter dialog.
The mother accommodates to the therapist, telling Morris not to inter-rupt. She has accepted the rule that people talk for themselves. The family sets are flexible, a sign of good prog-nosis.

Mrs. Gorden: Wait. Let me talk to her. So you got the chemistry set and started messing with it.

Mandy: Yes.
Mrs. Gorden: And you got the matches because you were trying to do an experiment.
Mandy: Yes.
Mrs. Gorden: Have you seen Morris light matches when he was doing it?
Mandy: No.

Mrs. Gorden: Well, why did you light a match? (*Mandy speaks inaudibly.*) What? (*Mandy mumbles again.*) She says that—well, Morris got a chemistry set for Christmas—and she always bothers with it. Because she bothers with everything. Everything! And he took it and put it in my room to keep her from bothering with it. So she asked to get this water. But instead of going downstairs, she went in my room to get the chemistry set. And she was trying to do an experiment. I don't know what kind she could have been doing with matches.

Montalvo: Mm.

Morris: An experiment I did—

Mrs. Gorden: Morris. Don't interrupt.

Montalvo: Is—I notice that—what's her name?

Mrs. Gorden: Joyce.

Montalvo: Joyce is very shy. Is she like that?

Mrs. Gorden: She is. All the time she's very quiet.

Montalvo: Very quiet? Joyce, did you see the mattress too?

Joyce: No.

Montalvo: No?

Joyce: No.

Montalvo: Where were you when it happened?

Joyce: In my room cleaning it up.

The mother amplifies Mandy's message for the therapist, acknowledging that he is participating in her dialog with Mandy. But although she again starts to talk with Mandy in an exploratory fashion, her tone of voice is harsh. The mother constantly blames Mandy. Mandy is afraid; she murmurs inaudibly. The mother's initial acceptance of the therapist's model for change and her reversion to her previous position are characteristic of all changing processes.

The mother has accepted the therapist's rule. She accommodates to the therapist, blocking Morris' interruption.

Ac. Maintains family structure by talking with the mother about the children and over their heads.

Re. Emphasizes weakness for the first time: Joyce's shyness. He is spreading the problem in order to change the original individual diagnosis into a family diagnosis.

Ac. Contacts fourth member. He talks with each member and expresses concern for all.

Montalvo: Who told you what happened? Did Mandy tell you what happened?

Ac. The therapist includes all the siblings and is respectful of the children's communication. His questions to them are concrete, requesting information on "how," which encourages a child's communication and makes him feel an important part of the session.

Joyce: She told me the clothes were on fire.
Montalvo: Did you get scared?

Re. Introduces concern for the child's affective experiences.

Joyce: No.
Montalvo: What did you do?

Re. Addresses child in terms of effectiveness. She could do something when she had to.

Joyce: I told Morris and then Morris came up. I told Morris the bed was on fire.
Montalvo: So. When you got home, you must have been pretty upset.

Re. Returns to Mrs. Gorden, respecting her function as head of the family and central communications switchboard. He expresses concern for her, following up his concern for the experience of a well sibling with the same concern for Mrs. Gorden. Again he is seeding. Later on, after concern has been accepted in the family system, he will introduce concern for Mandy. *Morris's functioning as a parental child makes him responsible for events that occur when Mrs. Gorden is out. He also seems to be her protector, taking on himself the responsibility for solving the crisis.*

Mrs. Gorden: Oh, well, when I came in, I smelled something burning and, well, Morris stayed up so he could tell me about it, so I walked in the door, and he—he said, "Mama, I've got to tell you something. You're going to be very angry." I said, "Well, first of all, why are you up? And what is that I smell burning?"
Montalvo: Did you try to find out what happened?
Mrs. Gorden: Yes, but she—this is the most I found out.

Montalvo: M-hm. Could you find out if she burned herself in any place?

Ac. Tracking, by expanding Mrs. Gorden's own knowledge of the fire.
Re. Moves Mrs. Gorden away from describing the event and back into enacting family transactions. Having listened and supported her, he knows he can now challenge her. He asks for dialog between Mrs. Gorden and Mandy with a statement of concern to which Mrs. Gorden complies perfunctorily. The therapist attempts to introduce a new affect (concern) by manipulating the content of the communication as well as its direction, from mother to child.

Mrs. Gorden: Did you burn yourself anyplace?

Mandy: No.

Mrs. Gorden: No, she didn't burn herself. I looked to see when I—

Montalvo: How about whether she was scared? It can be a pretty scary thing.

Re. Supports the identified patient. He does not accept the information given by Mrs. Gorden, because he is interested in the enactment of dialog with the affect of concern. He moves from concern about physical pain to concern about psychological pain. His previous seeding, first with Joyce and then with Mrs. Gorden, facilitates this approach.

Mrs. Gorden: Yes, she was—

Montalvo: Could you check?

Re. Insists on the enactment of transactional patterns.

Mrs. Gorden: Were you afraid?

Mandy: Yes.

Mrs. Gorden: You were afraid after it started burning.

Mandy: Yes.

Mrs. Gorden: You just don't know why you did it.

Mandy: No. (*She begins to cry.*)

Mrs. Gorden: Huh?

Mandy: No!

Mrs. Gorden: Well, you knew better, didn't you?
Mandy: Yes.
Mrs. Gorden: Because it's not the first time you did it, right?

Scapegoating behavior reasserts itself, despite the therapeutic maneuver. There is a long history of action and reaction to previous hurts that resists the therapist's modifying input.

(Later in the session. Mandy has been reading quietly.)

Montalvo: By the way, Mandy seems to love reading. Is that so?
Mrs. Gorden: I don't know. I'm not even sure she's reading that book.
Montalvo: Why don't we find out. Why don't you find out. Could you do it. Could she read for you?

The therapist returns to Mandy in a neutral area of current interaction.

Ac. Tracking an event, the girl's reading, and transferring it into an enactment of transactional patterns.
Re. Uses a task to frame the mother-child interaction.

Mrs. Gorden: Well, can you read this book?
Mandy: Yes.
Mrs. Gorden: Is this your reading book in school?
Mandy: M-hm.
Mrs. Gorden: All right. Read it. *(Mandy reads.)* I can't hear you.
Mandy (reading): "The Gingerbread Boy. This is the little old woman. . . ." *(She continues reading.)*
Montalvo: What do you think of that?
Mandy: ". . . I will make a gingerbread boy to eat. And she did."
Mrs. Gorden: Mandy, where did you leave off in school? You have already read this, right? Where did you leave off in school?

Mrs. Gorden again perceives the therapist and Mandy as a coalition against her and again attacks the junior member of the coalition. The pervasiveness of the dysfunctional scapegoating set may be owing to Mrs. Gorden's sense that the therapist has shifted his affiliation and is again sup-

porting Mandy. Mrs. Gorden attacks Mandy, first because she does not know how to read, then because "she read instead of paying attention."

Mandy: When I got to the end.
Mrs. Gorden: To the end.
Mandy: M-hm.
Mrs. Gorden: Well, what were you doing? Just reading it over again? Looking through it, or what?
Mandy: Reading it over.
Mrs. Gorden: Why are you reading it? Why aren't you paying any attention?
Montalvo: I'm sorry, what was that?
Mrs. Gorden: I asked her why was she reading the book; why wasn't she paying attention.
Montalvo: She was reading okay.

The therapist defends Mandy. He and Mrs. Gorden are now involved in a power operation in which Mandy is a pawn. In this operation Mrs. Gorden is invested in Mandy's failure. She admits Mandy's competence as if it is her own defeat because the therapist supports Mandy. The therapist is gaining experiental knowledge of family structure. The same sequence—therapist affiliating with Mandy; Mrs. Gorden attacking Mandy—occurred before, but it did not have the intensity needed to change the therapist's behavior. Now he apprehends the fact that Mrs. Gorden transforms direct support of Mandy into a coalition of Mandy and the therapist against her. He may have a hunch that he is re-creating a previous family structure that existed when the father was a permanent member, and he may store this hunch for future testing. But at the moment, he is experiencing resistance to support for Mandy. He must incorporate this experience into his therapeutic behavior.

Mrs. Gorden: Well, this she has already read.

Montalvo: Okay. And you wanted to test whether she could read further?

Mrs. Gorden: Yes.

Montalvo: Why don't you find out whether she can?

Mrs. Gorden: Where's the end?

Mandy: Here. That page.

Mrs. Gorden: This is the end?

Mandy: M-hm.

Mrs. Gorden: You know what this is?

Mandy: M-hm.

Mrs. Gorden: Can you read that? Have you already read it?

Mandy: No.

Mrs. Gorden: Can you read it?

Mandy: Yes.

Mrs. Gorden: Read it.

Mandy (reading): "The Three Bears. Once upon a time three bears lived in the woods. One bear was Father Bear. One bear was Mother Bear."

Montalvo: Okay, Mandy! Okay!

Mrs. Gorden: Well, she can read that all right.

Montalvo: But look. Look, I'll show you: "Yeah, she can do that. Yeah." What's going on with you?

Mrs. Gorden: What do you mean what's going on with me?

Montalvo: Almost anything that— she does a lot of good things. You know, she can read pretty good. She's friendly. You must have done a lot with her. Because she's not so far behind in reading or anything like you say.

Mrs. Gorden: Not—well, no, she's not far behind.

Montalvo: Yes.

Re. Reinforces his previous task.

Re. Mimics Mrs. Gorden's way of talking and acting. He attacks Mrs. Gorden directly because of her insistence on critical behavior.

Re. Modifies his attack on Mrs. Gorden by stating that Mandy's positives are a reflection of good mothering. This mixture of criticism with praise enables Mrs. Gorden to accept the criticisms, yet leaves her unable to defend herself.

Mrs. Gorden: It's just that I can't constantly be around her all the time. Like if I leave her upstairs and I go downstairs to do something, in two minutes somebody's calling me, something she did.

Montalvo: Who's calling you? Morris?

Mrs. Gorden: No, not only Morris.

Montalvo: Who?

Mrs. Gorden: Joyce, Debbie—all of them.

Montalvo: The last time that something like that happened, what was it?

Mrs. Gorden: Maybe like—when I send them upstairs, I say clean your room. So these two are supposed to be cleaning the room. Mandy, she doesn't do anything unless I'm standing there. Joyce will come down and say, "Mom, Mandy says she's not doing nothing." And if I go up there, Joyce might be straightening shoes up, but Mandy's messing them up. Joyce is hanging something up, she's taking it down.

Montalvo: You did a nice job, Mandy, on the reading. We forgot to tell her she did a nice job.

Mrs. Gorden: Yeah. Very good.

Montalvo: See, I'm concerned that— sure, we go around trying to find out. And I'm sure there are things that must be done so you feel safe when you're out. She will not do things like that when you're out. But you know, I'm a little bit more concerned with finding that Joyce is kind of shy. It's not just Mandy. Joyce is kind of shy and doesn't talk, and I see Mandy kind of scared.

Mrs. Gorden insists on not accepting the positives of Mandy. This may be one of the ways she responds to the therapist.

Re. Deflects a scapegoating attack by changing content, altering affect, and introducing other family members.

The siblings blame Mandy, agreeing with Mrs. Gorden. At this point in family life, Mandy is an easy target. When the siblings as well as the mother blame, the scapegoat's self-perception as the guilty one is reinforced.

Ac. The "we" invites the mother to join the therapist.

Re. Changes content, focusing on an area in which Mandy is competent.

Mrs. Gorden complies with the therapist, perhaps because by praising Mandy she can re-ally with him.

Re. Moves away from the focus on Mandy to look at both sisters and their affective lives. He has used this strategy at various times during the session. It seems effective for a while, then the focus on Mandy as the only family problem reappears.

Mrs. Gorden: No, she's not scared of me. She's probably frightened now about what—this is the way I feel. I feel that she's frightened because of what happened the other night. But she's not afraid of me. Now she will say more to me than Joyce will—things that happen. Or she'll come and talk to me about what happened today in school or things that happened. But Joyce never tells me things that happen in school.

Montalvo: Well, she's not scared, you say, and she does talk to you. You're right, those are good signs. Do you have any hunches as to what's happening that she will do these things that are prohibited and are things that should not be done?

Mrs. Gorden: Well, about that, I can't get anything from her. But she did say to Morris one time that she would like to go live with her father because he would let her do anything she wanted to. Well, when he was there, he says I'm mean to her because I won't let her do what she wants to. But he don't correct them right. Like if they do something, so, they just do it. He doesn't want them to get any whippings, you know, or be punished for anything. Now, Debbie, she's spoiled rotten. And like she is now— she used to be so terrible, you couldn't take her anywhere cause you'd be so embarrassed. And like now, one time Jerry took her out—when he was coming around, he doesn't come around at all now—and they went shopping or something. So I say I'm going to leave her with a babysitter because I don't want to take her be- cause I know how she acts when she's

Mrs. Gorden accepts the therapist's spreading of concern and includes Joyce as a problem. While the strategy of emphasizing positives in Mandy was thwarted a number of times, the therapist's use of the usual pattern of "concern" was accepted by the mother and Joyce was included.

Mrs. Gorden brings in problems of control with other children as part of her fight with her husband. It appears that husband and wife fought out their conflicts in the parental sphere. The father was seen as coalescing with the children against the mother. One can surmise that Morris and the mother versus the father and Mandy were cross-generational coalitions.

with you. But he said, "I want her to go." So I let her go. So we got in the store—it was a drugstore, I had to get some things. And she wanted something in there. And I said, "Well, Debbie, you can't have it." And she just stretched out on the floor and started kicking all the bottles of lotion off the shelf and all. Well, Jerry didn't want me to beat her. "Don't beat her. Wait till you get home. Wait till you get home." Then—

Montalvo: Was it the same way with Mandy?

Mrs. Gorden: No. She never acted like that.

Montalvo: I mean, did you and Jerry have a lot of things about—

Mrs. Gorden: Oh, well, he didn't want me to say anything to her.

Re. Explores the use of the children as detourers of husband-wife conflict.

Montalvo: I see. So there was a lot of problem between you and Jerry about the kids? He didn't want you to say anything to them.

Mrs. Gorden: No. He didn't want them to be corrected. So—

Montalvo: Who was Jerry's favorite? (*The mother points.*) Mandy? I thought so. I am wondering if—do you go to work tonight?

Re. Explores coalition across generational boundaries and makes implicit interpretations of Mandy's part of a Father-Mandy coalition against the mother.

Mrs. Gorden: Tonight? Yes.

Montalvo: At what time, around?

Mrs. Gorden: Well, I told them that I would be late.

Montalvo: I would like you to go home and to get the chemistry set. And Morris can go and take care of Joyce and Debbie for a while. And I would like you to take Mandy and teach her how to handle matches without burning herself or how to put fires out. You can take some of the small

Re. Sets a task for home. The task is framed only for two members. A different task is given to the other members, which will leave Mrs. Gorden and Mandy alone. The task is described in detail with familiar terms, in a positive mood. It is a play for Mrs. Gorden and Mandy alone, and Mrs. Gorden is put

pieces of paper and do it only till she is comfortable. If she cries, you don't play. Okay?

Mrs. Gorden: Okay.
Montalvo: Don't do too much. Do you have one of these egg timers? Kitchen timers for cooking?
Mrs. Gorden: Yes.
Montalvo: Do it only for ten minutes, no more than that. You could do it for ten minutes. Do you know, Mandy, what Mommy's going to do with you? Listen to this, Morris, because you are going to have to be taking care of Joyce and Debbie. This is only for Mandy to play. You cannot play, and you cannot play. Okay? You are the only one who can play with Mom. Mommy's going to teach you how to play with matches so that you don't get burned and so that you don't burn things. Okay? Will you teach her all you know? Will you teach her all you know about—you know how to light them? (*He is kneeling next to Mandy, patting her arm.*)
Mandy: Yes.
Montalvo: Will you teach her how to do that?
Mandy: Yes.
Montalvo: Okay. Teach her everything you know. Okay? Now I would like you to hold Mommy's hand. Okay? Now Mommy's going to teach you how to play with matches so that you don't get hurt and you don't hurt anybody. Okay?
Mandy: Yes.

in a position of giver to Mandy. These features of the task are designed to create a context in which the mother and scapegoated child can meet in a situation unusual in the family. Mrs. Gorden is competent, and Mrs. Gorden gives to Mandy; Mandy receives and accepts help from the mother.

Re. Ensures Mandy's cooperation by describing the task as a play in which she has a special part. Having gotten Mrs. Gorden to accept the task, he can talk directly to Mandy and model nurturant behavior toward her while assigning a task that may become stressful. He emphasizes that Mandy has competence and is to exercise that competence on her mother's behalf. The task supports Mrs. Gorden's centrality, but is directed toward creating a new style of interacting for Mrs. Gorden and Mandy.

Re. Uses physical contact to reinforce his task. He creates closeness and positive affect around a content dealing with achieving skills and avoiding pain.

Montalvo: Only ten minutes, though. Okay?

Re. Puts a limit on the task because he knows that prolonged contact between Mrs. Gorden and Mandy may result in more friction.

Mandy: Yes. (*Mrs. Gorden lets her hand go.*)

Montalvo: Okay. You know, I would like to see this family weekly. Can you keep this time? Maybe we can go at this very slowly. Because it looks to me like if—there are many other things here that I don't understand at all. Maybe you can help me, you know, understand what's happening. I am as concerned for Joyce, quite frankly, as you are for Mandy, though clearly this thing that happened with Mandy is very important, because the house could have burned down. But there is something of your having to get in there when you're not there, you know. There is no way out. You have to teach Mandy to take care of herself better.

Re. Toward the end of the session, makes the problem definitely a family problem.

The interview lasts five more minutes. The therapist reopens the husband-wife area, indicating that this will be part of the sessions. He tells Mrs. Gorden to be very sheltering toward Mandy during the ten minutes of the task. He asks the mother to call him the next day to tell him how the task went, and he tells her she may call him at any time. She snaps at Debbie, and he tells her that sessions can help her to be less nervous and tense with the children. The mother agrees that she would like to work around this area.

Following is a portion of the second interview with the same family, one week later. The therapist begins by asking Mrs. Gorden if she would like coffee. He compliments her on her appearance, compliments Joyce for always looking happy, and asks the mother how long it takes her to get the children dressed in the morning. The therapist thus initiates the session by acting as host, making the family comfortable. He is also responding to the family's mood (mimesis).

Montalvo: Mandy looks so different today. So happy.

The therapist takes responsibility for the transition into the session.

Mrs. Gorden: She's a little different today. I guess she was—last week, I guess she was kind of—you know, upset about what happened.

Mrs. Gorden has accepted the therapist's modeling. Her description of Mandy emphasizes the child's affect.

Montalvo: How did you do? I thought it was very nice, what you told me over the phone.

Ac. Supports Mrs. Gorden and highlights the continuity of their relationship.

Mrs. Gorden: Yeah. Well, what happened, what she was doing, she had the pack open. And she'd just strike the match. She's left-handed. So she's doing it all backwards anyway.

Montalvo: Let me see. Mandy, show me your left. (*She raises her left hand.*)

Ac. Makes contact with Mandy in an age-appropriate communication.

Mrs. Gorden: And she'd just strike toward the matches and light up the whole pack, you know. And it—I guess it kind of burned her, a little bit, so she dropped it—threw it.

Mrs. Gorden's description is related to competent implementation of the task. She now describes Mandy's fire setting as an accident or lack of competence instead of as malevolence.

Montalvo: Apparently you did a good job, you know, sensing what was wrong and teaching her.

Ac. Links Mandy's improvement to Mrs. Gorden's competence, maintaining the family structure of Mrs. Gorden's centrality.

Re. Links Mrs. Gorden and Mandy in a subsystem that is rewarding for Mrs. Gorden, changing the previous scapegoating transactions. He reinforces the new transactions.

Mrs. Gorden: M-hm.

Montalvo: Do you feel confident now that she knows how to handle it better?

Mrs. Gorden: Yeah, much better. (*She smiles happily.*)

Montalvo: Really?

Mrs. Gorden: Yeah.

Montalvo: Well, how many—there was a lot of practice there? You did a lot of practice with Mama?

Ac. Supports Mandy, emphasizing the work together.

Re. Supports the new subsystem through the junior member as well.

Mandy: Yes.

Montalvo: Yeah? How often?

Mrs. Gorden: Well, I did it every day. Sometimes I—

Mrs. Gorden responds to the therapist's support by describing how competently and effectively she responded to the task.

Montalvo: Every day!

Ac. Responds by being very pleased with both of them, and both feel satisfied with themselves; there is a spread of good feeling (mimesis).

Mrs. Gorden: M-hm. Sometimes I had time to do it twice before I went to work between the time she got home and the time that I left. But most days I only did it once.

Montalvo: No more than five minutes, I hope.

Mrs. Gorden: No. No.

Montalvo: I was wondering if—would you—could you light a fire for me?

Re. Uses the symptom to de-emphasize it. He has made the interpretation through the task that the fire setting was the result of a dysfunctional set in which Morris, the parental child, interrupts transactions between Mrs. Gorden and Mandy, with the development of scapegoating. Now he moves the enactment of fire setting within the context of the newly defined Mrs. Gorden-Mandy subsystem. The success of the task will support the positive bond between subsystem members.

Mandy: Now?

Montalvo: A good one? Just like Mommy taught you? Okay. Here. You do it right there. Okay. Now let me see. Can she do a good job? You will help her, okay? Without burning yourself, huh? Okay. Why don't you get closer to her so that you can help her. *(Mrs. Gorden and Montalvo change seats. Mandy lights a fire in an ashtray.)*

Montalvo: Okay!

Re. Maintains new family structure, decreasing the distance between Mrs. Gorden and Mandy, making Mrs. Gorden the helper.

Mrs. Gorden: Don't let the paper fall on the floor, because it will catch something on fire.

Montalvo: M-hm. That's a pretty good one. Would you know how to turn it off—would she know?

Ac. Supports Mrs. Gorden as central switchboard.
Re. Starts to guide Mandy, but stops himself and lets Mrs. Gorden take the guiding function.
Mrs. Gorden is imitating the therapist's modeling.

Mrs. Gorden: How would you stop that fire from burning?

Mandy: With water.

Montalvo: Very good. You see—

Mrs. Gorden: Well, would you—after you light the fire, would you go get the water, or what?

Mrs. Gorden facilitates exploratory behavior on her own.

Mandy: I'd get the water before I'd start the fire.

Montalvo: It's like this party you're going to. You need a man before you go to play cards. You can't be in there just by yourself. She needs water before she can get the fire out. Can I—Morris, why don't you get some water for her. You know where it is?

Re. Introduces a theme from the mother's life as an adult separated from her children. This is seeding, which will be amplified later.
Ac. Supports family structure, using Morris as a helper.

Morris: M-mm.

Montalvo: Can he get some water for you? Mandy?

Re: Supports Mandy's right to determine when she needs help.

Mandy: Mm.

Montalvo: Okay. (*To Morris*) I'll tell you where it is. Tell you exactly where it is. (*To Mrs. Gorden*) You can help her to find out what to do with the ashes. Maybe she should check to see that—you know—there is nothing burning. (*He leaves with Morris.*)

Re. Feels that Morris now needs support and goes with him to bring water. He accepts Morris' helping Mandy and also keeps Mrs. Gorden involved with Mandy. At the same time, the enactment of the task keeps the Mrs. Gorden-Mandy subsystem supported.

Mrs. Gorden: You have to check to know that there's nothing burning. How would you do that?

Mrs. Gorden facilitates Mandy's exploration. She is now imitating the therapist's modeling in his absence.

(*Later in the session.*)

Mrs. Gorden: I don't trust any of them with matches. I don't—

Montalvo: But she's (*indicating Mandy*) in better shape.

Re. Supports the differentiation of family members. He separates Mandy from a statement that puts all the children in the same category.

Mrs. Gorden: Yeah.

Montalvo: She's in much better shape. You have done your job with her.

Re: Reinforces previous statement by tieing Mandy's behavior to Mrs. Gorden's action, thereby directing Mrs. Gorden to support Mandy's individuation as competent.

Mrs. Gorden: I have never seen Joyce with any—but if she had them, striking them, I don't think she would do it right.

Montalvo: Well, why don't we do it here, just on that paper. Sure, Joyce.

Mrs. Gorden joins the therapist by exploring Joyce's behavior. She also describes Joyce as incompetent.

Re. Develops a task of setting a fire similar to the previous one, but he changes the cast, for the label of incompetent has shifted from Mandy to Joyce. Now Joyce will learn and Mrs. Gorden and Mandy will teach. This task moves Mandy from the position of learner to teacher, increases the strength of affiliation between Mrs. Gorden and Mandy, and increases Mandy's power in the sibling subunit.

Mrs. Gorden: Joyce.

Joyce: Mm?

Mrs. Gorden: Let me see you light a fire.

Montalvo: She's got to be the teacher. Mandy's got to be the teacher.

Mrs. Gorden: You have to show her what to do.

Montalvo: Hey, Mandy. You've got to show her what to do. Mama said. Now you show her—explain to her that she should show her in such a way that Joyce doesn't get burnt in any way. Okay?

At this point, the mother and therapist are a team.

Re. Supports Mandy in her new position, using the previous language of helping and care.

Mrs. Gorden: Show her so—listen to me. You know how I showed you so you won't get burnt. And I explained to you. Right? Can you explain to Joyce just like I explained to you?

Mrs. Gorden expands on the same theme that the therapist used. She delegates to Mandy in the same way that the therapist delegated her to teach Mandy. This delegation changes the previous structure, in which only Morris was the helper.

Mandy: Mm.
Mrs. Gorden: Let me hear you explain to her! Don't strike the match, but just explain to her.
Mandy (to Mrs. Gorden): You put—
Mrs. Gorden: Talk to her.

Mrs. Gorden short-circuits her own function as switchboard. Again her intervention is strikingly similar to previous therapeutic interventions. She directs Mandy to enact a dialog with Joyce. On resuming her executive function, Mrs. Gorden delegates.

Mandy: I don't know how.
Montalvo: Mama can help you.
Mrs. Gorden: You—she gets the matches, right? What does she do with them?
Mandy: Then you get some water. And put the water on the table, in a glass. And strike the matches, let them burn on some paper or something.

Mrs. Gorden and Mandy are imitating the previous mother-therapist dyad, while the therapist recedes and withdraws. Mandy is using longer sentences. Her teaching is very clear.

Mrs. Gorden: Well, why do you get the water?
Mandy: So if they catch onto anything you pour the glass—
Mrs. Gorden: You get the water and put it out. Right. Uh, well, about the match, in striking the match, what do you do?
Mandy: You tear a match off, then you close the book of matches up and light it.
Montalvo: Maybe she can show— maybe Joyce can do exactly the same thing.
Mrs. Gorden: Joyce, you know what

Re. Assigns a task.

she tells you to do? What did she say to do? (*Joyce speaks inaudibly.*) Yeah, well, you have the water. (*Joyce again mumbles.*)

Montalvo: Go ahead, Mandy, show her. I'm sorry. I interrupted you.

Mandy: You get the paper and put it on top, so it won't burn the table.

Montalvo: Can I put one in there, and you can light it up? You could show Mandy. I'm sorry. Here. Here's one. And here's two. Now. Really help her. Okay? Just like Mommy said. Really help her to light it up. And watch out for her fingers, 'cause she doesn't know how to close the thing too good. So you teach her how to do it good.

Ac. Directs Mandy, but is careful to underline Mrs. Gorden's teaching, as though he is operating by Mrs. Gorden's proxy. Under this mantle, he again speaks the language of care.

Mrs. Gorden: And after she strikes the match, how does she hold it?

Mandy: Up like this.

Mrs. Gorden: Up like what?

Mandy: This.

Mrs. Gorden: Out.

Mandy: Hold it out like this.

Mrs. Gorden: Right. Come over here, by the ashtray, and light that match. Show her how.

Morris: You don't strike it in your hand like that. (*Morris tries to help Joyce by showing her how to strike a match.*)

Montalvo: Morris, you're out of a job. Hey Morris, come over here, Morris. This guy works so much for you.

Ac. Contacts Morris, who has been displaced from his centrality and who therefore needs special support.

Re. Decreases the distance between himself and Morris, using the Montalvo-Morris dyad to move him out of the Mrs. Gorden-Morris dyad.

Mrs. Gorden: Right.

Montalvo: Relax, man. You have a vacation now. Okay? (*He moves Morris to a chair near him.*)

Re. Relabels his direction for change as a "gift" for Morris, relabeling Morris' previous help as overburdening him.

Mrs. Gorden: Go back over there.

Montalvo: Go over here, so that they can do it by themselves. You know, they've got to learn how to do it by themselves. Because sometimes—you cannot be all the time looking at them, taking care of them all the time.

Mrs. Gorden: You don't know where to strike it at? On this flat part.

Montalvo: She can ask Mandy too.

Mandy: On here.

Montalvo: That's true.

Mrs. Gorden: What's the matter?

Joyce: I don't want to.

Mrs. Gorden: You don't want to.

Montalvo: Be careful. Take your time. She's—you're not sure yet? She's not really sure of the grip, you see. Could you do one, so she sees how to do it, Mandy? Watch Mandy do it first. Real carefully. Take your time. (*Mandy lights the match.*)

Morris: M-hm.

Mrs. Gorden: You didn't light the other match.

Montalvo: Very good. Pretty good. Mandy, maybe Joyce shouldn't do it till she's ready. You see, because Mandy has had a lot of training. You really took your time with her. And you know, you did a lot of practice. Now, maybe when you teach Joyce, Mandy should be watching and teaching. Because I think she has good hand control now. The fingers are working real nice. Let me see something. Is it lit? Do it again. Close it again. That's very smart. That's very good. Now, do you have some rules in relation to that? Do you have some rules in relation to matches in the house and all that? I don't know. You told me you were going to.

Ac. Supports Morris' position as Mrs. Gorden's helper, talking to him as the other responsible member.

Re. Relabels: "helping" is "letting them do things themselves."

Ac. Accepts Joyce's fears.

Re. Insists on enactment of task and directs Mandy to finish it.

Re. Supports Mandy's new functions, but protects Joyce by making Mandy's competence the result of her interaction with Mrs. Gorden (supporting the Mrs. Gorden-Mandy dyad). The therapist then expands the dyad, giving directions for a Mrs. Gorden-Mandy-Joyce triad—a subsystem of women, which will exclude Morris and the baby. He contacts Mandy again in concrete ways, increasing proximity and body contact between them, modeling for the mother.

Mrs. Gorden: Yes. I have put them all up, so they don't know where they are. If I'm there, I might have cigarettes laying there, but I don't leave matches laying around.

Montalvo: That's the only one. Okay. Fine.

Re. Supports reality control.

Mandy's fire setting disappears after the first session. The therapist remains in contact with this family for a year and a half, until the mother moves back to the town where her family lives. He works intensively with the school to develop a program for Mandy to help her become more competent in that context. The school assigns her to one of its best and most sympathetic teachers. She blossoms under the positive attention at both home and school, and becomes much happier and more competent.

After the mother becomes ill, several sessions are held in the home. On one such visit, the therapist finds that the mother has suddenly been hospitalized and the children are being cared for by an elderly neighbor. He arranges for a homemaker to care for the children while Mrs. Gorden is in the hospital and during her first few days back at home. He sends her a plant, which seems to convey a symbolic message of nurturing and growing roots.

The therapist also works to free Morris from his excessive duties as a parental child. But when Morris begins to make friends in his peer group, the family is faced with Philadelphia's gang problem. Shortly afterward, the mother moves away. Each year she sends the therapist a Christmas card and a picture of each of the children. A follow-up two years after the initiation of therapy shows that the family is still functioning adequately.

This case illustrates other aspects of a therapist's job. Although changes within a family can be effective, to be lasting, such changes cannot be achieved in isolation from a family's circumstances. Working with the family in its context is essential to modifying and then perpetuating the modifications.

12 A Longitudinal View: The Browns and Salvador Minuchin

The kind of interview dealt with so far has been a therapist's or consultant's initial meeting with a family. In this situation, joining techniques and other aspects of different therapists' styles are most easily spotted. To discuss what happens in therapy after the initial interview is more difficult. The drama of immediate interactional patterns fades, and attention is increasingly given to the bolder strokes required to achieve the desired outcome. Nevertheless, a study of family therapy would not be complete without a look at the overall therapeutic process, as provided in the case of the Browns.[1]

The Browns were referred to therapy by a pediatrician treating their daughter, Sally, aged ten. Sally had been hospitalized with the diagnosis of anorexia nervosa, a psychosomatic syndrome whose main symptom is an extreme weight loss because of failure to eat. Sally had lost fifteen pounds in ten weeks. On her arrival at the hospital she weighed forty-two pounds; after a week there, she weighed forty pounds. She looked like an emaciated old woman, with a sad, fixed smile.

Sally's family is composed of her father, who is a successful architect in his mid-forties, her mother, and three siblings—Michael, aged fourteen, Robert, aged twelve, and John, aged eight. They assess themselves as a "normal American family," whose only severe problem is Sally's refusal to eat. They came into family therapy only because the pediatrician insisted.

240

According to Hilde Bruch, the syndrome of anorexia nervosa, is characterized by a disturbance of delusional proportions in a person's concept of his own body; a disturbance in his perception, or cognitive interpretation, of stimuli arising in his body, with a failure to recognize signs of nutritional need as its most pronounced deficiency; hyperactivity and a denial of fatigue, which is another manifestation of the falsified awareness of one's bodily state; and a paralyzing sense of ineffectiveness, which pervades all thinking and activities.[2]

Treatment designed according to this theoretical orientation would involve a variety of procedures, including dietary regulation, medication, and psychodynamic therapy or behavior modification. All these techniques are directed primarily toward the individual patient, the "container" of the illness.

A family therapist approaches anorexia nervosa from a different angle. A psychosomatic symptom, like other symptoms, can be the expression of a family dysfunction in the identified patient.[3] The symptom may be the patient's attempted solution to the family dysfunction, as was the case with the Smiths. Or it may have arisen in the individual family member because of his particular life circumstances and then been utilized and supported by the family system as a system-maintaining mechanism. In any case, it is inconceivable for the family therapist to regard the identified patient as separate from his circumstances. Treatment procedures are directed toward the identified patient within his family.

The concept of the identified patient changes when the individual is seen as an acting and reacting member of a social system regulated by an implicit structure. The illness is no longer confined to him. Although his symptoms are the most evident expression of a problem, his particular illness is at best only a partial truth. Illness has developed within the life context. In effect, the individual's symptoms have been made the figure, while everything else has been made ground. But as treatment evolves, other family members' behavior and interactions will become the figure, temporarily carrying the burden of being "symptomatic." The goal is to change the system, in an atmosphere that emphasizes interdependency, mutuality, and support.

THE PSYCHOSOMATOGENIC FAMILY MODEL

The therapeutic approach to the Brown family is guided conceptually by the model of a "psychosomatogenic family."[4] This model was developed in the course of experiences with many families in which the identified patients had widely differing psychosomatic and psychogenic symptoms. Accordingly, the interventions of a therapist using this model are not limited merely to his own responses to current family transactional patterns. As he joins the family, he has a model to guide his probes, against which he can test the idiosyncratic circumstances of the particular family. According to this conceptual model, the development of psychosomatic illness in a child is related to three factors. They include a special type of family organization and functioning, involvement of the child in parental conflict, and physiological vulnerability.

The kind of family functioning involved is characterized by enmeshment, overprotectiveness, rigidity, and a lack of conflict resolution. In enmeshment, the family members are overinvolved with one another and overresponsive. Interpersonal boundaries are diffuse, with the family members intruding on each other's thoughts, feelings, and communications. Subsystem boundaries are also diffuse, which results in a confusion of roles. The individual's autonomy is severely restricted by the family system.

In an overprotective family, its members have a high degree of concern for each other's welfare. Protective responses are constantly elicited and supplied. When there is a sick child, for example, the entire family becomes involved. Often conflicts are submerged in the process. The child in turn feels responsible for protecting the family.

Rigidly organized families often present themselves as not needing or wanting any change in the family. Preferred transactional patterns are inflexibly maintained.

Finally, the lack of conflict resolution in a family means that it has a low threshold for conflict. Some families simply deny the existence of any conflict. In others, one spouse is a confronter but the other is an avoider. Others bicker, but manage to avoid a real confrontation. Consequently, issues are not negotiated and resolved. The psychosomatically ill child plays a vital part in his family's avoidance of conflict by presenting a focus for concern. The system reinforces his symptomatic behavior in order to preserve its pattern of conflict avoidance.

The involvement of the child in parental conflict is the second characteristic of the typical psychosomatogenic family. In families in which the boundaries between the spouse subsystem and the children are diffuse, the sick child is particularly important in detouring spouse conflict. When submerged or unnegotiated conflicts threaten the spouse dyad, the identified patient is brought in (and indeed, brings himself in), to form a rigid triad.

The physiological vulnerability of the child is a necessary but not sufficient component in the appearance of a psychosomatic syndrome. For example, the appearance of psychosomatically triggered attacks in a diabetic child depends on the existence of the other elements of the psychosomatogenic family. The presence of physiological vulnerability in anorexia nervosa is debatable.

THE BROWN FAMILY DIAGNOSIS

The diagnostic model of the psychosomatogenic family helps the family therapist to approach a case of anorexia nervosa. But as always, the road between the formulation of goals and the attainment of those goals will be traversed by the family and the therapist in a unique way, dictated by their idiosyncratic joining. It is sometimes useful to work with families with an anorectic child by developing crises, organizing the family's transactions in such a way that it is forced to deal with the stresses it has been submerging. The therapist monitors the resulting crises, creating experiential situations in which the family members can and must learn to deal with each other in new and different ways.

The Browns, for example, insist on defining themselves as "perfectly normal" except for one member's medical problem. In this situation, a medically induced crisis may open up the significance of the family transactional patterns that have created and supported the symptom. The symptom area offers the obvious route to this crisis.

The transcript that follows begins as the family, including all four children, and the therapist sit down at a lunch table, which has been set up in the therapy room. The session began at 11:00, and after the initial stages of the interview, the family was asked to order lunch.

The technique of eating with an anorectic family is valuable for several reasons. For one thing, it makes things happen in the session with the therapist. When the conflict around eating can be reenacted in the session, merely to talk about food would represent a waste of time. Furthermore, organizing a family crisis around the symptom makes the symptom available to direct intervention. Interventions on an individual level directed at exploring the anorectic's ideas about food and eating might serve only to reinforce and further crystallize the symptom. But when a *family* crisis is organized around the syndrome, it is not the symptom itself but the interpersonal negotiations of parents and child around eating that gain salience. Not to eat becomes the ground instead of the figure as a result of the dramatic emergence of interactional factors, which then become available for interventions to produce change.

In the Brown family, the therapist begins to develop a crisis in the family by telling the family members that it is essential for Sally to eat. Having eaten almost nothing except ice cream, she has been losing weight rapidly. Now she must eat to survive. The therapist asks the family to order lunch. Sally refuses to order anything but ice cream and cake, so the therapist tells the parents to order for her. They agree on ordering a hamburger, commenting that she has always liked hamburgers.

This everyday scene of the struggle for autonomy and control sets the stage for a family crisis. The session is conducted at a high pitch of emotion. Sally is crying, screaming, and sometimes hitting. The mild parents, who prize the avoidance of conflict in their family, suddenly find themselves in the midst of a conflictual transaction that they cannot escape. As has been characteristic of the family, the parents disqualify each others' request to Sally, with the result that she cries in despair but does not eat. The therapist then instructs the father alone to make her eat.

Minuchin: She must eat, so I want you, Mr. Brown, to help her.

Mr. Brown: You can have the ice cream after you eat.

Sally: I am not eating! I am not eating it! I am not eating it! (*She gets up and runs to a corner of the room, crying.*)

Mrs. Brown: She wanted a coke and she got milk.

Mr. Brown: I'll get you a coke tonight, all right? (*He gets up and goes after Sally.*)

Mrs. Brown: Did you ask for coke?

Minuchin: Yes, she did.

Mr. Brown: Don't worry about it, I promise you I will give you coke tonight. Now don't cry, Sally. (*She pushes him away.*) Do you think I have a coke? Come on, Sally.

Mrs. Brown: Do you want something else?

Mr. Brown: She can get real mad at me again. (*He tries to lead Sally back to the table; she resists.*)

Sally (screaming): I hate him! I hate him! I hate you, sir.

Mr. Brown: Who do you hate, Sally?

Sally: Him.

Mr. Brown: Who, the doctor?

Sally: I don't like him!

Mr. Brown: He's a nice guy.

Sally: I don't like him!

Mr. Brown: All right.

Sally: The doctors at the hospital let me have what I wanted. Not him. I don't want to be here. I just want the ice cream. I just want the ice cream!

Mr. Brown: You can have the ice cream after you finish the hamburger.

Sally (screaming): I'm not having the hamburger.

Mr. Brown: Why not?

Sally: I don't want it! (*She sobs uncontrollably.*)

Mr. Brown: Well, quit crying, quit crying.

Sally: I don't want it. I don't want it, Daddy.

Mr. Brown: You have always liked hamburgers before. (*He puts his arms around her.*)

Sally: I did not. Now leave me alone, I don't want it. I don't want the hamburger, I just want the ice cream. Let go of me! (*She pushes him.*)

Mr. Brown: Why are you so mad?

Sally: I just want the ice cream. I don't want the hamburger. Will you get off of me?

Mr. Brown: The only way to get rid of the doctor is to eat.

Sally: I am not having it, I am not having it, I am not having it, I am not having it, I am not having it! (*Mr. Brown gives up and sits down. Sally remains in her corner. The three boys are crying.*)

Minuchin: Could you help her eat, Mrs. Brown?

Mrs. Brown: I don't know, but I don't have patience like his. (*She gets up and moves toward Sally.*)

Sally (screaming): I am not having it, I am not having it!

Mrs. Brown: Sally, it's for your own good. Please. Please honey.

Sally: No, I won't.

Mrs. Brown: Don't you want to get well?

Sally (shrieking): I am not doing it. Oh, shut up! I am not eating it!

Mrs. Brown: Don't you want to go home?

Sally: I am not eating it, I am not eating any food here.

Mrs. Brown: We would like you to.

Sally: I am not.

Mrs. Brown: I would like you to.

Sally: I am not going to. (*She slaps her mother.*)

Mrs. Brown: Don't hit me. Don't hit me, I said!

Sally: I am not going to!

Mrs. Brown (sharply): Don't hit me, I said! I would like you to eat.

Sally: I am not going to.

Mrs. Brown: Why not?

Sally: I am not going to.

Mrs. Brown: Do you want to disappear?

Sally: I don't have to. I want to go back to the hospital.

Mrs. Brown: You can't go back to the hospital until you eat your lunch. Does it make you happy to hit me? Are you happy hitting me? Are you happy?

Sally: Yes, because then you won't bite me.

Mrs. Brown: I won't bite you.

Sally: I just want ice cream.

Mrs. Brown: And we want you to eat.

Sally (screaming): I don't care, I am not having it.

Mrs. Brown: Do you want me to scream back at you?

Sally: I don't care. I am not having it, I am not having it, I am not going to have it, I am not eating it! (*She sobs and stamps her feet.*)

Mrs. Brown: I hope you're happy now that you made me unhappy.

Sally: I am not eating it.

Mrs. Brown: Would you please come to dinner.

Sally: I am not eating it, I am not eating it!

Mrs. Brown: Why not?

Sally: Leave me alone.

Mrs. Brown: Why won't you—

Sally: Leave me alone!

Mrs. Brown (to Minuchin): Am I supposed to keep going?

Minuchin: Sally, you'll have to sit down.

Sally: I just want the ice cream!

Mr. Brown: First sit down. (*Sally refuses.*)

Sally: I am not eating it!

Minuchin: Sit down. (*He gets up and points to a chair. Sally sits down.*)

Sally's sitting down marks the beginning of a new stage in the session. The whole family is exhausted and searching for a way out of the rigid dysfunctional pattern in which they feel trapped. The therapist offers a model of negotiation. He suggests alternative selections of food, among which Sally must decide. By choosing from them, Sally is making decisions about the management of her life in the hospital and her eating arrangements there. During the session, the therapist poses approximately forty alternatives. Sally makes eleven decisions, and each time the therapist supports her competence. She obviously enjoys feeling that she has some control over her environment.

This strategy of offering alternatives is shown in the next segment, which is a dyadic interaction between Sally and the therapist, with the help of a pediatric resident who acts as the therapist's deputy. The parents' attempts to intervene are blocked, resulting in a separation between Sally and her parents and the creation of a therapeutic dyad—Sally and the therapist.

Minuchin: Sally must eat. It is not a question that she has an option. She must eat. Now the question is that you can eat something that you want instead of something that you don't want, but this will need to be with the doctor's approval. So tell him what kind of foods you like because you will need to eat. Tell him what kind of foods you like.

Sally: I don't know.

Minuchin: You will need to tell him because he will ask the kitchen for the kind of food you will get. Decide the ones that you like more. Which ones do you like most?

Mr. Brown: Well—

Minuchin (gesturing for silence): No, no. It is Sally. It is her eating and it is in the hospital, and this is something we need to handle now.

Sally: I don't know.

Minuchin (To resident): What kind of foods does she need to have?

Resident: Fish, some meat.

Minuchin (to Sally): Oh, so let's start with that. In what form do you want your meat?

Sally: I don't know.

Minuchin: Well then he will serve it to you in any way that the kitchen gives.

Sally: Okay.

Minuchin: Would you like to deal with this doctor exclusively? You know, you can stop here and make an agreement with the doctor when you are alone. Do you prefer that or do you want to do it here? (*She nods.*) He says you need to have meat. What other things does she need to have?

Resident: Vegetables.

Minuchin: What kind of vegetables do you like? Tomatoes? (*She shakes her head.*) What other vegetable?

Resident: They probably have just about anything. Peas, string beans, spinach.

Minuchin: Which ones do you want?

Sally: Peas.

Minuchin: Do you have any other vegetable that you like? Peas, would that be okay? (*She nods.*) So we have meat and peas. Do you want chicken? Do you want chicken or meat?

Sally: Chicken.

Minuchin: Okay, so you get chicken. Fried or broiled? How do you want the chicken?

Sally: I don't know.

Minuchin: Is it okay fried, or do you want it broiled?

Sally: I don't know.

Minuchin: It's the same? So we have chicken, peas, What else does she need?

Resident: Starch—potatoes or noodles.

Minuchin: What do you like?

Sally: Neither.

Minuchin: What else?

Resident: Dessert.

The strategy of offering alternatives yields immediate results. Sally starts eating during the session, continues to eat during two more days in the hospital, and keeps eating after her return home. In a month she returns to her previous weight.

Once the dramatic presenting symptom, with its reifying characteristics, has disappeared, Sally and the rest of the family members appear considerably more complex. At the same time, the family map becomes clearer and more differentiated. As always, broadening the focus exposes the forces within the family that have been maintaining the apparent problem, which makes them susceptible to intervention.

The therapist's assessment of the Brown family is that they are operating in a tightly enmeshed system. Dyadic transactions rarely occur; interaction is either triadic or group. It is characterized by a rigid sequence, which promotes a sense of vagueness and confusion in all family members. For example, if a parent criticizes one of the children, the other parent or a sibling will join in to protect the child, and then another family member will join the critic or the criticized.

The original issue becomes diffused, only to emerge again later in a similar sequence and to be similarly unresolved.

The Brown family's enmeshed interactions have a helpful, protective quality. Their avoidance of aggression or even disagreement is striking. The family itself describes all its interactions as harmonious. Yet in the therapist's assessment, there are many unnegotiated husband-wife conflicts. Such conflicts have been submerged and never allowed to become explicit. They are expressed in the family organization, in which the mother has joined the children in a coalition that traps husband-father in a position of helpless isolation. He is perceived by the mother and children as an absolute despot, but in reality, his power within his family is negligible. The mother parents the children; the husband-father remains disengaged and peripheral. Only in the area of parenting are spouse disagreements expressed. The father feels that the mother is too lenient.

Another expression of disagreement that may be related to the selection of the anorexia symptom appears in the mother's constant attempts to improve the father's table manners. This disagreement has run throughout the twenty years of the marriage and is now discussed with bantering by all the family members, particularly at mealtime.

The boundaries of the spouse subsystem are very weak. The peripheral husband-father has strong ties to extrafamilial systems, particularly his business and his own family of origin. The mother is firmly bound in the mother-children subsystem, which is an enmeshed, highly resonant system. The mother is the main point of contact between this subsystem and others. As a result, the father communicates with the children through the mother. Because the mother controls the nature of such communication, she screens out its nurturant elements but lets in controlling elements, strengthening the coalition between herself and the children against the father. Her relationship with the children is overcontrolling, intrusive, and overnurturing. The close communication, appropriate with younger children, has led to difficulties, which started a number of years before when the older son, emerging into adolescence, began to make demands for the increased autonomy appropriate to his age. At the time of therapy, the relationship of the mother and oldest son is fraught with his demands for autonomy, countered by her demands for obedience. The middle brother is allied with his older brother in this conflict.

The family malfunctioning has affected all the family members.

Although the symptoms of anorexia nervosa have overshadowed the problems of the parents and the "well" siblings, clinical scrutiny of the total group shows that each member is responding to family stress in idiosyncratic ways.

The anorexia nervosa syndrome has been deeply imbedded in the family's pathogenic transactional patterns, making it unusually resistant to change. When a situation that requires change occurs, the family typically insists on retaining its accustomed methods of interaction. Consequently, situations of chronic imbalance are maintained for long periods, with Sally functioning as the chief conflict-detouring pathway. Her most important source of reinforcement is in the spouse subsystem, but the symptoms are multidetermined, finding reinforcement in both the sibling subsystem and the self.

Within the spouse subsystem, the never-negotiated conflicts between the parents are perceived as a particularly dangerous area. Although all the children are involved in keeping these conflicts submerged, it is most often Sally who crosses the generational boundary to diffuse the parental conflict. Her function is to allow her parents to detour their conflict via their concern for her.

Furthermore, the symptom defines a "safe" area in which spouse conflicts can surface. The father thinks the mother should make Sally eat, whereas the mother, while worried, thinks that Sally should not be forced to eat. The coalition of the mother and daughter against the father is explicitly manifested in the mother's protection of Sally against her father's assertion that she should eat. At the same time, Sally's selection of this symptom represents an implicit coalition with her father, whose fight with the mother has also been allowed to surface in the area of eating, namely, his table manners.

Within the sibling subsystem, Sally is the least powerful member of a rather undifferentiated group. She is isolated and excluded. The sibling subgroup conforms to the family style. Whenever conflict arises, there is an immediate bunching in coalitions. Sally is always excluded from these coalitions, and is often their target. Yet since open disagreement must be avoided, her isolation takes the form of a withdrawal into her musical interests. The anorexia nervosa keeps this structure of the sibling subgroup intact, while also improving Sally's position. She remains isolated, but the center of concern and protectiveness.

For Sally herself, the anorexia syndrome is a means of self-assertion. By not eating, Sally is asserting herself in a way that is permissible within the value system of the family. She is disagreeing, but not openly. The family's priority of avoiding conflict is maintained, because her failure to eat is not an explicit confrontation or rule breaking.

The symptom, then, is being reinforced by all the family members. The spouses accept it as a conflict-avoiding circuit, and one spouse uses it in coalition against the other. Sally experiences it as a form of permissible self-assertion, as well as a means to protect her family and even ally, on an implicit level, with her father. The siblings also reinforce the symptom as part of a protective and scapegoating system.

THERAPEUTIC GOALS

As a result of this diagnosis of the Brown family transactional patterns, five therapeutic goals can be formulated. First and foremost is the disappearance of the anorexia nervosa syndrome.

Second, a transformation must be effected in the spouse subsystem. This will require that supportive, complementary transactions between the spouses be increased, so as to create a clearly bounded subsystem of the mother and father, parenting their children in a mutually supportive relationship. The mother must also be disengaged from parenting, to give her more space for spouse subsystem operations. And the father's engagement in parenting must be increased, to enable him to contact his children directly without going through their mother. The mother's function as contact, in other words, must disappear.

The third goal of treatment is a transformation in the sibling subsystem. The enmeshed functioning of the subsystem must be decreased, and the boundaries opened, so that the children can interact with their parents and with the extrafamilial world without choosing a representative of their needs. Moreover, there must be increased autonomy appropriate to their age for all the children and a change in Sally's powerless, scapegoated position.

The fourth goal of therapy in this case is to make possible the formation of effective dyads and triads in the total family system. The degree of flexibility within the subsystems must be increased, and enmeshment decreased. Flexible alliances and coalitions must be possible.

Clear communication among all family members must be fostered. In this way, the real nature of their transactions can be recognized.

These objectives are of course mutually interdependent. Any effective transformation is predicated on the possibility of restructuring at least two family members within the family organization. Furthermore, the goals are interlocked within the system, just as is the pathology. The older sons cannot become adolescents until the mother becomes a wife. The mother cannot function as a wife until her husband pulls her away from the children. The mother will not let the children go until the father offers her support and tenderness as a husband. As long as contact between the father and children takes place only via the mother, the father and mother cannot move into their own spouse orbit. While the mother and father remain divided, the children must continue to struggle with the mother's intrusive overnurturance and overcontrol. As long as the children remain part of an undifferentiated, highly enmeshed sibling subgroup, they will continue to struggle with the mother by using the anorectic sibling, which further reinforces the syndrome.

THERAPEUTIC STRATEGIES

From these therapeutic goals, specific strategies must be evolved to effect the necessary restructuring. The core of the Brown family's problems is the inability of the spouses to negotiate with each other. Accordingly, spouse subsystem sessions are held as the family therapy continues. Once the facade of mutual agreement has been broken, the spouse sessions deal with the wife's sense of being unacceptable to her husband, her feeling of being in competition with her mother-in-law, her complaints about her husband's failure to support her in parenting and to respect her as an adult. The husband brings up issues of his isolation in the family, of his inability to scold his children except at his wife's direction, and of his wife's lack of interest in him as a sexual partner. Therapeutic interventions in these subsystem sessions are addressed to facilitating the negotiation and resolution of disagreements and encouraging the experience of mutually supportive, pleasurable, nonparenting interactions.

Concurrently, sessions with the whole family are continued. Various strategems are utilized during these sessions. For example, the family's style of communication is challenged. When a conflict between two members develops, the therapist makes them continue until they have achieved a resolution or until a third member has joined the argument in an explicit form, either by asking to be included or upon being invited by the original dyad. Members of the family change their chairs so as to permit the two or three people involved in a discussion to sit next to each other; the others move out of the circle and observe.

This technique is particularly useful in differentiating the siblings from each other. For example, as the oldest boy's conflicts with the mother become prominent, the father is requested to intervene. The three bring their chairs to the center of the room, while the other children move out. With the mother being strongly supported by her husband, negotiations ensue that permit Michael much more autonomy, explicitly related to his status as the oldest. The therapist increases this differentiation by treating him in an adult manner. He also assigns a task to the mother. She is to watch for actions that Michael performs which deserve her approval, and reward them. This strategy is directed to a dual audience, for Michael, who also hears the task assignment, increases the type of actions that his mother can reward. Michael begins to emerge as a teenager.

The individuation and disengagement of Michael from the sibling subsystem leaves twelve-year-old Robert the playmate of eight-year-old John; Sally, aged ten, is excluded. Now the three younger children are asked to occupy the center of the room, with the mother and father helping them from outside the circle. John and Robert are directed to play with Sally. But when the three play a board game together, the game becomes enmeshed and chaotic. Therefore, the children are assigned the task of playing board games at home. The parents are to buy the games and then see that the rules of the game are followed.

Robert, the brightest and most psychologically minded of the family, begins to ally with the therapist, sitting near him and commenting on the family's functioning. He begins to have more school friends and spends more time with them in an age-appropriate process of contacting the extrafamilial. Sally and John grow closer.

In one session, John complains that Sally plays roughly and frightens him with her fury. Now John and Sally take to the center of the room, with Michael asked to come and act as the mediator, helping John to understand Sally's explanation of her behavior. His role as oldest brother is buttressed by participation in an activity that differentiates his two youngest siblings. In all these family sessions, the clear demarcation of the parties in a negotiation and the resolution of clearly stated conflicts are emphasized.

The use of space to create actual proximity and distance, delimit subgroups (actors and observers), intensify affect, or potentialize the enactment of fantasies or roles is useful in rigid, highly enmeshed and undifferentiated families. It enables the therapist to function like the director of a play, setting the stage, creating a scenario, assigning a task, and requiring the family members to function within the new sets that he has imposed.

Therapy with the Brown family terminates successfully after nine months. The presenting problem has stopped being a family concern within a month of the initiation of therapy. A follow-up a year and a half after termination shows that the family is now involved in the typical difficulties of effectively functioning families and is coping with them satisfactorily.

Restructuring strategems, such as the interventions made with the Browns, can best be conveyed by describing family members and the therapist as though they were cybernated robots. Despite the obvious inaccuracies of this approach to describing human beings or therapy with human beings, it is the only way in which almost a year of complicated human transactions within a therapeutic system can be communicated according to the linear rules of logical exposition.

The therapeutic work with the Brown family is very different from work with the Smiths, the Dodds, and the Gordens. Each therapeutic system is in fact unique. Within the different contexts, therapist and family members always have different experiences. But underneath all this diversity, there are rules, because as Giovanni Guareschi noted: "The basic problems of my family are the same as those of millions of families; they spring from a family situation based on the necessity of adhering to the principles that are the foundation of all 'ordinary' homes."[5] Moreover, the number of possibilities of joining in human situations is finite, as is the number of strategies within the therapeutic system. Human limitations create a finite number of possible social structures. Perhaps in the future, therefore, a more systematic description of families and of family therapy can be developed.

Epilog

Scientific inquiry generally begins by marking off a specific area for investigation. Thereafter, the investigator restricts his view to that limited area, excluding other subjects. The region artificially segregated for study is in effect a creation of the investigator, for in reality it must always be a part of a larger field, with which it interacts. As John Spiegel stated: "We can no longer afford, in any science, to focus exclusively on one region and to leave the rest of the universe out of account until we complete our investigations. We never actually 'complete' our investigations, the nature of science being a continuous process of inquiry. Completeness is an illusion; and if, in any one science, we forever keep the rest of the universe out of account, we will never be in a position to consider the whole."[1]

This book has concentrated on family therapy. To include the entire family as a factor in mental health enlarges the perspective from the traditional concentration on the individual apart from his social context. Yet even this focus distorts the view of the psychological field, for it ignores the linkages between family and society.

According to the suggested model, an effectively functioning family is an open social system in transformation, maintaining links with the extrafamilial, possessing a capacity for development, and having an organizational structure composed of subsystems. The individual, who is himself a subsystem of the family, faces different tasks and acquires different interpersonal skills in the different subsystems.

255

Although to treat the family as a whole may simplify the task of relating the individual to his social context, it may also distort one's view of any particular individual in the family. Clearly, not all changes in the family affect all its members, and changes in one member do not necessarily affect all other members in the same way.

However, the model of an effectively functioning family suggests directions for family therapy. From it the therapist can derive a structural map of the troubled family, which helps him delineate specific goals for therapy. The therapist then joins the family in a therapeutic system with the intent of restructuring it in a defined way. His joining maneuvers ensure the participation of family members in the therapeutic process, as well as their cooperation in enhancing the family's own healing functions. The therapist's restructuring efforts either facilitate the maintenance of subsystems that promote healing and growth, or help to form new subsystems which will achieve these ends.

Although different therapists might agree on a therapeutic goal for a particular family, their techniques for achieving that goal will vary. Therapists, having individual personalities and skills, develop idiosyncratic ways of relating. They can use themselves better if they learn to know and accept their own styles.

Talmudic treatises start on page two, to indicate that they are never complete. By the same logic I was tempted not to print the last page of this book. Clearly, by selecting and framing data on family therapy, I have created an artificial boundary around the family and the therapist. It is impossible to do otherwise.

Further Readings
Notes
Index

Further Readings

The following suggested readings offer additional information on the processes of joining and restructuring in family therapy, as described in Chapters 7 and 8.

Ackerman, Nathan W., ed. *Family Therapy in Transition.* Boston, Little, Brown, 1970.

———. *Treating the Troubled Family.* New York, Basic Books, 1966.

Auerswald, E.H. "Interdisciplinary vs. Ecological Approach," *Family Process*, 7 (1968), 202-215.

Beels, C.C., and Ferber, A.S. "Family Therapy: A View," *Family Process*, 8 (1969), 280-310.

Bell, John E. *Family Group Therapy.* Public Health Monograph #64. Washington, D.C., Department of Health, Education, and Welfare, 1961.

Bloch, Donald A., ed. *Techniques of Family Psychotherapy: A Primer.* New York, Grune & Stratton, 1973.

Boszormenyi-Nagy, Ivan, and Framo, James L., eds. *Intensive Family Therapy.* New York, Harper & Row, 1965.

———, and Spark, Geraldine. *Invisible Loyalties.* New York, Harper & Row, 1973.

Bowen, Murray. "Perspectives and Techniques of Multiple Family Therapy," in Bradt, J. and Moynihan, C., eds. *Systems Therapy.* Privately published by Bradt and May, Washington, D.C., 1971.

Duhl, Frederick J., Kantor, David, and Duhl, Bunny S. "Learning, Space, and Action in Family Therapy: A Primer of Sculpture," in Bloch, Donald A., ed. *Techniques of Family Psychotherapy: A Primer.* New York, Grune & Stratton, 1973.

Framo, James L., ed. *Family Interaction: A Dialogue Between Family Researchers and Family Therapists*. New York, Springer, 1972.

Friedman, Albert S., *et al. Family Treatment of Schizophrenics in the Home*. New York, Springer, 1965.

Haley, Jay, ed. *Changing Families: A Family Therapy Reader*. New York, Grune & Stratton, 1971.

_____. *Strategies of Psychotherapy*. New York, Grune & Stratton, 1963.

_____. *Uncommon Therapy: The Psychiatric Techniques of Milton H. Erikson*. New York, Norton, 1973.

Haley, Jay, and Glick, Ira D. *Family Therapy and Research: An Annotated Bibliography of Articles and Books, 1950-1970*. New York, Grune & Stratton, 1971.

_____, and Hoffman, Lynn. *Techniques of Family Therapy*. New York, Basic Books, 1967.

Jackson, D.D., and Lederer, W.J. *Mirages of Marriage*. New York, Norton, 1969.

Kaffman, Mordecai. "Short Term Family Therapy," *Family Process*, 2 (1963), 216-234.

Laing, R.D., and Esterson, A. *Sanity, Madness and the Family*. London, Tavistock, 1964.

Langsley, D., and Kaplan, D. *The Treatment of Families in Crisis*. New York, Grune & Stratton, 1968.

Laqueur, H.P., *et al.* "Multiple Family Therapy: Further Developments," *Int. J. Soc. Psychiat.*, special edition no. 2 (1961), pp. 70-80.

Macgregor, R., *et al. Multiple Impact Therapy with Families*. New York, McGraw-Hill, 1964.

Minuchin, Salvador, *et al. Families of the Slums: An Exploration of Their Structure and Treatment*. New York, Basic Books, 1967.

_____. "Family Therapy: Technique or Theory?" in Masserman, Jules H., ed. *Science and Psychoanalysis*, vol. XIV. New York, Grune & Stratton, 1969.

_____. "The Plight of the Poverty-Stricken Family in the United States," *Child Welfare*, 44 (1970), 124-130.

_____. "The Use of an Ecological Framework in Child Psychiatry," in Anthony, E. James, and Koupernik, Cyrille, eds. *The Child in His Family*. New York, Wiley, 1970.

_____, and Barcai, Avner. "Therapeutically Induced Family Crisis," in Masserman, Jules H., ed. *Science and Psychoanalysis*, vol. XIV: *Childhood and Adolescence*. New York, Grune & Stratton, 1969.

Patterson, G.R., Ray, R., and Shaw, D. *Direct Intervention in Families of Deviant Children*. Oregon Research Institute, Eugene, 1969.

Paul, N.L. "The Use of Empathy in the Resolution of Grief," *Perspect. Biol. Med.*, 11 (1967), 153-169.

Rubenstein, D. "Family Therapy," *Int. Psychiat. Clin.*, 1 (1964), 431-442.

Satir, Virginia. *Conjoint Family Therapy*. Palo Alto, Science and Behavior, 1964.

Speck, Ross, and Attneave, C. *Family Networks*. New York, Pantheon, 1973.

Watzlawick, P., *et al. Pragmatics of Human Communication: A Study of Interactional Patterns, Pathologies, and Paradoxes*. New York, Norton, 1967.

Whitaker, Carl A., and Miller, M.H. "A Reevaluation of 'Psychiatric Help' When Divorce Impends," *Amer. J. Psychiat*, 126 (1969), 57-64.

Wynne, Lyman C. "Some Indications and Contraindications for Exploratory Family Therapy," in Boszormenyi-Nagy, Ivan, and Framo, James L., eds. *Intensive Family Therapy*. New York, Harper & Row, 1965.

Zuk, Gerald. *Family Therapy: A Triadic-Based Approach*. New York, Behavioral Books, 1971.

————, and Boszormenyi-Nagy, Ivan. *Family Therapy and Disturbed Families*. Palo Alto, Science and Behavior Books, 1967.

Notes

1. STRUCTURAL FAMILY THERAPY

1. José Ortega y Gasset, *Meditations on Quixote* (New York: Norton, 1961), p. 104.

2. John Milton, *Paradise Lost*, I, 254-255.

3. Ortega, *Meditations on Quixote*, p. 45.

4. Gregory Bateson, "The Cybernetics of Self: A Theory of Alcoholism," *Psychiatry*, 34 (1971), 1.

5. José M.R. Delgado, *Physical Control of the Mind: Toward a Psychocivilized Society* (New York: Harper & Row, 1969), p. 129.

6. *Ibid.*, p. 132.

7. *Ibid.*, p. 243.

8. Delgado's concept must be broadened to include the neurovegetative system, as Neal Miller's work demonstrated, and the endocrinal system, as in Selye's investigations.

9. Aaron T. Beck, "Paranoia," mimeo, University of Pennsylvania. Used by permission of the author.

10. Erving Goffman, "Insanity of Place," *Psychiatry*, 32 (1969), 357-358.

11. See Margaret J. Rioch, "All We Like Sheep—(Isaiah 53:6): Followers and Leaders," *Psychiatry*, 34 (1971), 258-273.

2. FAMILY DEVELOPMENT

1. Giovanni Guareschi, *My Home Sweet Home* (New York: Farrar, Straus, and Girous, 1966), pp. vii-viii.

262

3. A FAMILY MODEL

1. Roger G. Barker, *Ecological Psychology: Concepts and Methods for Studying the Environment of Human Behavior* (Stanford: Stanford University Press, 1968), p. 6.

2. Nicholas S. Timasheff, "The Attempt to Abolish the Family in Russia," in Norman W. Bell and Ezra F. Vogel, eds. *A Modern Introduction to the Family* (Glencoe: Free Press, 1960), pp. 55-63.

3. Phillip Aries, *Centuries of Childhood* (New York: Vantage Press, 1962).

4. R.D. Laing and Aaron Esterson, *Sanity, Madness, and the Family* (London: Tavistock, 1964).

5. Salvador Minuchin, "Adolescence: Society's Response and Responsibility," *Adolescence*, 16 (1969), 455-476.

6. Ivan Boszormenyi-Nagy and Geraldine Spark, *Invisible Loyalties* (New York: Harper & Row, 1973).

5. THERAPEUTIC IMPLICATIONS OF A STRUCTURAL APPROACH

1. Claude Lévi-Strauss, *The Scope of Anthropology* (London: Cape, 1967), 25-26.

2. Salvador Minuchin, "The Use of an Ecological Framework in the Treatment of a Child," in E. James Anthony and Cyrille Koupernik, eds. *The Child in His Family* (New York: Wiley, 1970), pp. 41-57.

6. THE FAMILY IN THERAPY

1. Jay Haley, "Family Therapy," in Alfred M. Friedman, Harold I. Kaplan, and Benjamin J. Sadock, eds. *Comprehensive Textbook of Psychiatry* (Baltimore: Williams and Wilkins, in press).

2. R.T. Sollenberger, "Why No Juvenile Delinquency?" paper presented at the American Psychological Association meetings, New York City, 1966.

7. FORMING THE THERAPEUTIC SYSTEM

1. Claude Lévi-Strauss, *The Scope of Anthropology* (London: Cape, 1967), pp. 26-27. *Italics mine.*

8. RESTRUCTURING THE FAMILY

1. Harry Aponte and Lynn Hoffman, "The Open Door: A Structural Approach to a Family with an Anorectic Child," *Family Process*, 12 (1973), 1-44.

2. "A Modern Little Hans," film available from Philadelphia Child Guidance Clinic.

3. A. Aichhorn, *Wayward Youth* (New York: Viking, 1935).

4. Ronald Liebman, Salvador Minuchin, and Lester Baker, "An Integrated Treatment Program for Anorexia Nervosa," mimeo., Philadelphia Child Guidance Clinic.

5. Salvador Minuchin et al., *Families of the Slums; An Exploration of Their Structure and Treatment* (New York: Basic Books, 1967).

6. Salvador Minuchin and Avner Barcai, "Therapeutically Induced Family Crisis," in Jules Masserman, ed., *Science and Psychoanalysis*, vol. XIV: *Childhood and Adolescence* (New York: Grune & Stratton, 1969), pp. 199-205.

7. Salvador Minuchin, "The Use of an Ecological Framework in the Treatment of a Child," in E. James Anthony and Cyrille Koupernik, ed., *The Child in His Family* (New York: Wiley, 1970), pp. 41-57.

8. Elie Wiesel, *Souls on Fire: Portraits and Legends of Hasidic Masters* (New York: Random House, 1970).

9. A "YES, BUT" TECHNIQUE

1. William H. Masters and Virginia E. Johnson, *Human Sexual Inadequacy* (Boston: Little, Brown, 1970).

12. A LONGITUDINAL VIEW

1. For this case, see also Salvador Minuchin, "Structural Family Therapy," in Gerald Caplan, ed. *American Handbook of Psychiatry*, vol. III (New York: Basic Books, in preparation).

2. Hilde Bruch, *Eating Disorders: Obesity and Anorexia Nervosa* (New York: Basic Books, 1973).

3. Salvador Munichin, Lester Baker, Bernice L. Rosman *et al.*, "Psychosomatic Illness in Children: A New Conceptual Model," mimeo., Philadelphia, Penna.

4. This model was developed during a research project whose participants are Salvador Minuchin, Lester Baker, Ronald Liebman, Leroy Milman, Bernice L. Rosman, and Thomas C. Todd, supported by the National Institute of Mental Health (MH 21336).

5. Giovanni Guareschi, *My Home Sweet Home* (New York: Farrar, Straus, and Giroux, 1966), p. viii.

EPILOG

1. John Spiegel, *Transactions: The Interplay Between Individual, Family, and Society* (New York: Science House, 1971), p. 38.

Index

accommodation, 122, 123, 124-125,
131, 133, 136, 139, Chs. 9-11
passim, 252
actualizing transactional patterns, 122,
140-143, 172-173, 219, 223, 243
adolescents, 50, 58, 64, 104, 126, 133,
135, 147, 155, 166, 168, 249, 252,
253
affect, 155, 182, 216, 217, 222, 223,
227
aged, therapy of, 11-12
Aichorn A., 154
"An American Family," 49
anorexia nervosa, 103, 104, 112, 122,
128, 145, 153, 154, 240-241. *See
also* Brown family
asthma, psychosomatically triggered,
13
autonomy: individual, 55, 59, 92,
144-145, 146, 156, 191, 216, 218,
242, 244, 247, 250; subsystem, 54,
56, 57, 59, 143-147

Baker, Lester, 7
Barker, Roger G., 48
Barragan, Mariano, 87

Bateson, Gregory, 5, 6
Beck, Aaron, 10
blocking transactional patterns, 92, 93,
94, 103-104, 147-148, 177, 220,
221, 247
boundaries, 53-56, 242, 249
boundary negotiation, 22-23, 30, 32,
41, 57, 101; therapeutic, 56, 57, 60,
94, 98, 100, 114, 118, 135, 136,
143-147, 170, 173, 197, 251
brittle diabetes. *See* diabetes, superlabile
broadening the focus, 3, 4, 13, 104,
105, 130, 132, 155, 159, 160, 166,
187, 191, 192, 194, 206, 209, 211-
212, 221, 227, 248
Brown family, 103, 145, 153, Ch. 12
Bruch, Hilde, 241

change: concept of, 91, 111, 136;
resistance to, 52, 110, 161, 176,
195. *See also* system maintenance
child rearing, 33-35, 44-45, 47-48,
57-58, 78-80, 95-96, 145, 200,
249, 252
coalition, 36-37, 61, 64, 94, 98, 99,

265

104, 111, 224, 225; stable, 102, 213, 228–229, 249, 250

communication. *See* transactional patterns

confirmation, therapeutic, 113, 121, 126, 127, 149, 156, 163, 170, 171, 187, 189, 194, 202, 222, 223, 234, 237

conflict resolution, 61, 63, 73, 148, 149, 242, 249

contract, therapeutic, 18, 96, 132–133, 140, 231

countertransference, 91

crisis induction, 104, 131, 156, 243, 244

Delgado, Jose, 5–6, 14

delinquency, 92, 154

depression, 1, 100, 117, 132, 154, 158. *See also* Smith family

detouring, 8, 94, 101, 102, 149, 229, 242, 250

diabetes, 7–9, 93; superlabile, 7–9, 103, 243

diagnosis, process of, 89, 109, 129–132, 136, 206, 208–209

disengagement, 54–56, 130, 144

divorce, 65, 100–101

Dodds family, 125, 128, 133, 143, Ch. 10, 254

drug abuse, 107

emphasizing differences, 148

enmeshment, 54–56, 113, 127, 130, 134, 144, 145, 149, 151, 156, 242, 248, 249, 251, 252

enuresis. *See* Dodds family

escalating stress, 147–150

existential group. *See* family therapist groups

extended family, 17, 18, 20–23, 32, 38, 62, 76, 83, 95–98, 112, 134, 147, 167–179, 188

extracerebral mind, 6, 7, 9, 111

extrafamilial: individual contact with, 17, 29–30, 39, 48, 57, 59, 61, 64, 65, 114, 157, 214, 249, 251; family contact with, 18, 46–47, 49, 50, 57, 62, 63, 69, 70, 82, 130, 207–208, 255

family, attacks on, 48–49

family structure. *See* system: family

family therapist groups, 136

feminism, 49, 115

fire setting. *See* Gorden family

Freud, S., 51

goal, therapeutic, 104, 111, 125, 150, 206, 212, 251–252, 256

Goffman, Erving, 10

Gorden family, 98, 125, 127, 134, 135, 142, 146, 148, 150, 151, 152, 155, Ch. 11, 254

Guareschi, Giovanni, 16, 254

Haley, Jay, 111

handicapped, 65

hero, man as, 4

identity, sense of, 14, 47–48, 53, 55, 113, 120

individual. *See* subsystem: individual

individual therapy, 2–3, 4, 9, 11, 91, 106, 112, 129, 131, 255

initial session, special tasks of, 206–212

intrapsychic. *See* individual therapy

introjection, 4, 91

Jiménez, 119

joining, 89, 91, 109, 111, 113, 122, 123, 130, 136, 138, 148–149, 155, 210, 240, 242, 243, 256

kibbutz, 48, 50, Ch. 4

Laing, R. D., 49

leader, therapist as, 111, 123, 139, 151, 212

Levi-Strauss, C., 90, 124

Liebman, Ronald, 112, 128

maintenance, 125–127, 212

manipulation, therapeutic, 139

map, family, Ch. 5, 124, 130, 147, 152, 206, 210, 248, 256

Masai, 50

Masters and Johnson, 188

migraine, 114

mimesis, 128–129, 165, 166, 171, 186, 195, 197, 231, 233

modeling, 169, 198, 202, 216, 220, 230, 232, 234, 238, 246

Montalvo, Braulio, 125, 126, 127, Ch. 11

mood. *See* affect

mutuality, interpretations of, 56, 120, 121, 149, 196, 199, 200

nonverbal communication, 42, 90, 92, 131, 140, 209

obesity, 13

ombudsman, 63

one-way mirror, 96, 135, 142, 147

open doors, family with, 127, 134, 145, 151, 156

Ortega y Gasset, 2, 4, 5, 6

overcentralization, 140

overprotection, 13, 242, 249

Paradise Lost, 4

paranoid thinking, 9-12

parental child, 97-98, 134, 135, 142, 151, Ch. 11 *passim*

parenting. *See* child rearing

Peary, parable of, 2, 12

phobia, 104, 105, 153

poverty, 63, 95, 156, 208. *See also* Gorden family

psychodynamic therapy. *See* individual therapy

psychogenic vomiting, 103, 154

psychosomatogenic family, 241-243

Puerto Rican family, 63

Rabin family, Ch. 4, 206

reality: experience of, 2, 11, 12, 13, 14, 15, 40, 89, 111; challenging experience of, 117, 160, 162, 165, 186, 187, 189, 203

relabeling, 155, 156, 167, 168, 201, 220, 237, 238

restructuring, 123, 131, 135, 136, 138, 152, 155, Chs. 9-12 *passim*, 252, 254, 256

rigid triad, 101-104, 113, 146

scapegoating. *See* Gorden family

schizophrenia, 106

school, therapist contact with, 4, 63, 157, 239

sexual relations, 17, 82, 114, 115, 127, 132, 145, 180-183, 188, 252

single-parent families, 105-106, 134. *See also* Gorden family

site of pathology, 3, 4, 9-12, 241

Smith family, 1, 126, 129, 141, 142, 143, 145, Ch. 9, 254

social context, 2, 3, 4, 5-12, 46, 130, 131; animal experiments, 5-6; physiological effect, 7-9

socialization. *See* child rearing

space, use of, 94, 122, 136, 142-143, 146, 150, 172, 177, 192, 220, 252

Spiegel, John, 255

spreading the problem. *See* broadening the focus

structural group. *See* family therapist groups

structure. *See* system: family

style, therapeutic, 120-122

subsystem: individual, 52, 106-107, 211, 255; parental, 17, 26, 33, 35, 54, 57-59, 96, 97, 99, 133, 142, 145; sibling, 59-60, 108, 113, 134, 135, 145, 146, 250, 252; spouse, 17, 33, 35, 56-57, 61, 99, 101-104, 114-115, 135, 145, 146, 170, 250, 251, 252

subsystems, 52, 53, 55, 133-136

suction, 114, 139, 148

symptoms: therapeutic focus on, 152-155, 233, 243; use in system, 110, 152, 241, 242

system: family, 14, 89, 110, 130, 151; family schema, 51, 66, 255, 256; therapeutic, 9, 90-95, 111, 115, 123, 129, 136, 139, 147, 150, 206-212, 254, 256

system maintenance, 52, 110, 162, 163, 167, 169, 173, 175, 176, 178, 180

tasks: family, 14, 15, 18, 46, 61, 88; therapeutic, in session, 92, 93, 150, 171, 176, 224, 226, 233, 244; therapeutic, at home, 118, 137, 151, 186, 214, 229, 253

Tavistock, 10

tracking, 127-128, 160, 192, 198, 218, 219, 223, 224

transactional patterns, 17-18, 51-52, 62, 66, 131, 140, 142, 152, 180, 184-185, 209, 248-249; formation of, 17-18, 19, 22, 27, 32, 52, 119

transference, 3, 114
transferential group. *See* family
  therapist groups
transformation, structural, 2, 13, 14,
  91, 111, 119, 187. *See also* restructuring
transition, family in: developmental
  changes, 17–18, 33, 52, 60, 63–65,
  99–105, 110, 115–117, 130;
  response to societal changes, 46–47,
  50

triangulation, 102

unit, therapeutic. *See* system: therapeutic

Wagner family, Ch. 2, 47, 48, 51, 57,
  62, 88, 206
Whitaker, Carl A., 125, 126, Ch. 10